GASTROINTESTINAL ENDOSCOPY

ADVANCES IN DIAGNOSIS AND THERAPY

Volume One

GASTROINTESTINAL ENDOSCOPY

ADVANCES IN DIAGNOSIS AND THERAPY

Volume One

Edited by

P. R. Salmon
*Consultant Physician and Senior Clinical
Lecturer in Gastroenterology
School of Medicine
University College London*

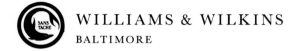

WILLIAMS & WILKINS
BALTIMORE

First published in 1984
© *1984 Chapman and Hall Ltd*

Distributed in Continental North, South and Central America,
Hawaii, Puerto Rico and The Philippines by
WILLIAMS & WILKINS CO.
by arrangement with
CHAPMAN AND HALL LTD

ISBN 0 683 07494 6

*Printed in Great Britain at the
University Press, Cambridge*

Library of Congress Cataloging in Publication Data

Main entry under title:

Gastrointestinal endoscopy.

   Bibliography: p.
   Includes index.
   1. Endoscope and endoscopy. 2. Gastrointestinal system
– Diseases. I. Salmon, P. R. (Paul Raymond)
RC804.E6G375 1984   616.3'307545   84-13075
ISBN 0-683-07494-6

Contents

LIST OF CONTRIBUTORS

D. J. Allison, MD, BSc, FRCR,
Consultant and Senior Lecturer,
Hammersmith Hospital and
Royal Postgraduate Medical School,
London, UK.

J. F. W. M. Bartelsman, MD,
Department of Gastroenterology,
Academic Ziekenhuis,
University of Amsterdam,
Amsterdam, The Netherlands.

L. H. Blumgart, BDS, MD, FRCS,
Director and Professor of Surgery,
Royal Postgraduate Medical School,
Hammersmith Hospital,
London, UK.

P. C. Bornman, MMed (Surg), FRCS,
Principal Surgeon,
Groote Schuur Hospital,
Cape Town, South Africa.

S. Braunfeld, MD,
Department of Medicine,
Mount Sinai Hospital,
New York, USA.

L. R. Celestin, MD, FRCS,
Consultant Surgeon,
Department of Gastroenterology,
Frenchay Hospital,
Bristol, UK.

D. G. Colin-Jones, MD, FRCP,
Consultant Physician and Gastroenterologist,
Queen Alexandra Hospital,
Portsmouth, UK.

J. D. Davies, MD, BS, MRCS, FRCPath,
Consultant Senior Lecturer in Pathology,
University of Bristol, and
Honorary Consultant and Head of
Histopathology Department,
Bristol Royal Infirmary,
Bristol UK.

L. Demling, Prof. Dr. med.,
Director, Medical Department,
University of Erlangen,
Erlangen,
West Germany.

D. A. W. Edwards, MD, FRCP,
Physician and Reader in Gastroenterology,
Faculty of Clinical Sciences,
University College,
London, UK.

P. Frühmorgen, Prof. Dr. med.,
Chief of Medical Department,
Ludwigsburg,
West Germany.

P. H. Harper, MA, MCh, FRCS,
Wellcome Research Fellow,
Nuffield Department of Surgery,
John Radcliffe Hospital,
Oxford, UK.

K. Huibregtse, MD,
Department of Gastroenterology,
Academisch Ziekenhuis,
University of Amsterdam,
Amsterdam, The Netherlands.

R. H. Hunt, FRCP, FRCP(C),
Professor and Head,
Division of Gastroenterology,
McMaster University Medical Center,
Hamilton, Ontario,
Canada.

T. Ihre, BA, MD
Associate Professor, Department of Surgery,
Södersjukhuset, Stockholm,
Sweden.

V. Jaffe, MA, MB, BCh,
Senior House Officer, Department of Surgery,
Hammersmith Hospital,
London, UK.

M. G. W. Kettlewell, MA, MChir, FRCS,
Consultant Surgeon,
John Radcliffe Hospital,
Oxford, UK.

R. E. Kirsch, MD, FCP(SA),
Associate Professor, Department of Medicine,
Groote Schuur Hospital and
University of Cape Town,
and Co-Director, Medical Research Council,
Liver Research Group,
Cape Town, South Africa.

M. J. S. Langman, MD, FRCP,
Professor of Therapeutics,
University of Nottingham Medical School,
Queens Medical Centre, Nottingham, UK.

W. Matek, Dr. med.,
Medical Department,
University of Erlangen,
Erlangen,
West Germany.

R. F. McCloy, BSc, MD, FRCS,
Senior Registrar, Department of Surgery,
Royal Postgraduate Medical School,
Hammersmith Hospital, London,
and Visiting Endoscopist to Her
Majesty's Prisons, UK.

F. G. Moody, MD,
Professor and Chairman,
Department of Surgery, Medical School,
The University of Texas
Health Science Center at Houston,
Houston, Texas, USA.

J. D. R. Rose, MA, MB, MRCP,
Senior Registrar,
Llandough Hospital, Penarth,
Glamorgan, UK.

P. R. Salmon, BSc, MB, FRCP, FRCP(E),
Consultant Physician and
Senior Clinical Lecturer in Gastroenterology,
School of Medicine,
University College London,
London, UK.

J. P. Schuppisser, MD,
Assistant Professor, Department of Surgery,
University of Basel,
Kantonsspital, Basel, Switzerland.

P. M. Smith, MD, FRCP,
Consultant Physician,
Llandough Hospital, Penarth,
Glamorgan, UK.

C. P. Swain, BA, BSc, MRCP,
Research and Honorary Senior Registrar
in Gastroenterology,
University College Hospital
and St. James' Hospital,
London, UK.

J. Terblanche, ChM, FRCS, FRS(SA),
Professor and Head of Surgery,
Groote Schuur Hospital and Somerset Hospital,
Cape Town; Professor and Head,
Department of Surgery,
University of Cape Town;
and Co-Director, Medical Research Council,
Liver Research Group, Cape Town,
South Africa.

P. E. Tondelli, MD, FACS,
Associate Professor, Department of Surgery,
University of Basel,
Kantonsspital, Basel, Switzerland.

G. N. J. Tytgat, MD, PhD,
Professor in Gastroenterology,
Head, Division of Gastroenterology,
Academic Medical Centre,
University of Amsterdam,
Amsterdam, The Netherlands.

C. W. Venables, MS, FRCS,
Consultant Surgeon in Gastroenterology,
Freeman Hospital,
Newcastle-upon-Tyne, UK.

J. D. Waye, MD,
Chief, Gastrointestinal Endoscopy Unit,
Mount Sinai Hospital,
New York, USA.

Preface

Over the past ten years a new dimension has been added to the study of digestive tract disease by the introduction and development of fibreoptic endoscopy. Throughout this period of time, quite rightly, considerable emphasis has been placed on the technology of fibreoptic endoscopes and their supporting systems and the need to train doctors to perform careful, skilful examinations. To this end a proliferation of books have appeared concentrating on these aspects. It should not be forgotten, however, that at the same time there have been enormous advances in imaging techniques, in interventional radiology and in the therapeutic demand and applications of flexible endoscopes. As a result of these changes, an annual meeting was convened three years ago by myself entitled 'Growing Points in Endoscopy'. These meetings have been sponsored by Pyser Ltd, UK distributors of Fujinon flexible endoscopes. The first four meetings have proved so successful that it was decided to produce a book encapsulating a number of important subjects highlighted by the meetings. The choice of material has entirely been my own and in no way attempts to cover the whole of digestive endoscopy. It is hoped however that this book will provide an insight into the rapidly changing and developing art and science of fibreoptic endoscopy and its expanding role as a therapeutic discipline.

P. R. Salmon

Section A

GASTROINTESTINAL HAEMORRHAGE

'The Difficult Bleeder – Recent Advances'

I

Endoscopic diagnosis

G. N. J. TYTGAT

Expertly performed endoscopy appears, in most instances, to offer the best available method for identifying the source of the bleeding lesion.

In principal, emergency endoscopy should be performed in any patient with upper intestinal bleeding and, in experienced hands, a firm diagnosis can be obtained in 80–90% of the patients. Endoscopy may not be applicable when bleeding is so massive that immediate surgery appears to provide the only hope of saving the patient's life. In this situation, endoscopy may be useful in the operating room to help the surgeon in locating the bleeding lesion.

The popularity of emergency endoscopy persists in spite of the fact that improved diagnostic accuracy has not yet been shown to improve overall patient survival. Indeed the mortality rate of around 10% has been unchanged for the past three decades [1, 2, 3]

THE ENDOSCOPIC PROCEDURE

Emergency endoscopy should be performed preferably in the endoscopy unit where all the necessary equipment is available. Many units have an emergency trolley set up each evening. If necessary this can be taken to the operating room or to the intensive care unit.

It is imperative that full resuscitative facilities are available together with skilled staff experienced in dealing with emergencies. Few units have specialized endoscopy nurses, available at night or during the weekends. As an alternative, intensive care nurses may be trained to assist during emergency endoscopy. Endoscopy should not take place until resuscitation procedures and any necessary transfusions are under way to correct hypovolemia. It is also wise to wait at least four hours after recent intake of food or barium.

A major debate has centred around the optimal timing for emergency endoscopy. When endoscopy is performed early it is usually possible to define the real cause of bleeding. Stigmata of recent bleeding may disappear within 24 hours. Varices or ulcers which have bled may look blameless 1–2 days later and by that time, an acutely ill patient may have developed acute gastric or duodenal erosions which may be interpreted erroneously as the original bleeding source. Forrest *et al.* [4] showed that bleeding lesions were found in 78% of the patients if endoscopy was carried out within 24 hours of admission but in only 32% if this was delayed to 48 hours. This was largely confirmed by the recent ASGE prospective bleeding study in which it was shown that early endoscopy offered the highest likelihood of finding an oozing or pumping lesion. The yield of actively bleeding lesions which was overall 32.6% increased to 41.5% when endoscopy was performed within the first 12 hours of admission. No increase in the incidence of active bleeding lesions was detected if the interval from admission to endoscopy was shortened to 3–6 hours [5]. Most units have evolved a compromise by which most bleeding patients are examined within 18–24 hours of admission. The majority of the examinations are fitted into the routine endoscopy lists within normal working hours, when the entire endoscopy team is present. However the availability of a skilled endoscopist on short notice for the most urgent problems, including nights and weekends, is mandatory.

Although many endoscopists perform urgent endoscopy without sedation, it is wise in an anxious patient to use some intravenous sedation cautiously. Most often diazepam is used [5].

Routine gastric lavage with iced, diluted saline solution before the endoscopy is not necessary because the endoscopic examination is hampered by massive amounts of blood in less than 5% of patients. In that case, the endoscope should be removed and reintroduced after performing lavage with a large bore multiple-holed tube (Ryle or Ewald tube). The quantities of fluid necessary for adequate evacuation of blood and clots vary greatly and often amount to at least two litres. There is no prospective study that shows that an attempt to induce local gastric hypothermia with iced fluid stops massive bleeding. Most would agree however, that it makes subsequent endoscopy easier and more informative. When bleeding stops, the return becomes clear. A small amount of coffee-ground material, small bits of old clots or slight pink discoloration are consistent with the cessation of significant bleeding. A clot may block the tube but this should not happen with proper lavage technique. Although suction should not be exerted via the tube lest confusing lesions be created for subsequent endoscopy, the lavage fluid should be injected with sufficient force to dislodge any clots that may be present. Drainage on the other hand should be by gravity. Occasionally the tube is localized to a small pocket which appears clear despite active bleeding distally. This artefact can be minimized by moving the tube back and forth. A large plastic 'overtube', placed over the endoscope prior to insertion is increasingly used. Once the instrument has passed into the stomach, the overtube is slid through the pharynx and past the cardia. If excess blood is encountered, it is easy to withdraw the endoscope leaving the overtube behind which facilitates the lavage procedure and the reintroduction of the fibrendoscope.

Since oesophageal lesions are common, a forward-viewing endoscope should always be used first. Rarely a side-viewing instrument may also be required. Small endoscopes are convenient in severely ill patients but their small suction channels are more easily obstructed by clots. Therefore standard foreward-viewing instruments are advised whenever possible.

Endoscopy should proceed with the patient in the left lateral position, preferably on a table which can be tilted head down. In the left lateral position, blood pools along the greater curvature of the stomach, which is fortunately an unusual area for bleeding lesions. Even with considerable quantities of blood in the stomach, it is usually possible to perform an adequate survey of the oesophagus, oesophagogastric junction, lesser curvature of the stomach, entire antrum and first two parts of the duodenum. Usually the oesophagus can be quickly examined for a bleeding source. One should quickly skim over the surface of a large pool of blood in the stomach, when present, and seek the pyloric opening in order to examine the duodenum. One should not waste time in the second portion of the duodenum unless blood is seen coming from it or when a rare postbulbar ulcer is suspected. Once the bulb has been exonerated, one can withdraw into the stomach and try to view different portions of the stomach. A U-turn manoeuvre is then performed, retroflexing the tip of the instrument and sliding it along the lesser curvature up to the fundus, allowing visualization of the entire fundus, cardia and oesophagogastric junction from below. It is not uncommon during the procedure that the patient evacuates large amounts of blood and clots by vomiting after which the lesion may become obvious. Even when a likely bleeding site has been detected, a complete survey should always be obtained because many patients have more than one lesion.

The presence of fresh blood may be of vital diagnostic importance. Minor diagnostic trauma is often inevitable and fresh blood is thus of significance only before the instrument has passed over the bleeding area. After visualization of a bleeding lesion, target jet irrigation with water or saline is applied to clear the lesion of adherent blood or clot. Irrigation can be performed by passing a tube through the biopsy channel although more sophisticated devices such as an irrigator-electrode canula or the recently introduced 'Bicap system' or the 'electro-hydrothermo' (EHT) probe are certainly easier to use. If the bleeding site is not identified in these circumstances and if there is a large collection of clotted blood along the greater curvature and in the fundus, it is then necessary to perform either gastric lavage or to turn the patient carefully with the scope in place onto his right side to complete the examination. This manoeuvre clears the fundus and upper greater curvature of clotted blood by allowing it to drop down into the lower body and antrum which have already been examined.

During endoscopy, intermittent oropharyngeal suction is performed by the nurse assistant to keep the patient's mouth clear of secretions and blood and to help prevent tracheal aspiration. At the end of the procedure after the scope is withdrawn, the patient is instructed to cough well to clear any tracheal secretions.

Usually in over 80% a complete examination is possible. The reasons for incomplete examination are excessive blood in the upper gastrointestinal tract, poor patient cooperation, technical difficulties, pyloric or duodenal deformity, limiting scope passage, retained food or antacids etc.

When an urgent diagnosis is required and the endoscopic view is persistently obscured by blood because of massive bleeding, then it still can be possible to give the surgeon useful information regarding the presumed site of bleeding. In certain circumstances for example it is only possible to demonstrate that the bleeding is not coming from the oesophagus, that a Mallory–Weiss laceration is excluded or that there is no evidence of aspirin-induced antral erosions. Furthermore the appearance of blood welling back into the stomach through the pylorus may be considered good evidence of a bleeding duodenal ulcer even if it is impossible to visualize the duodenal bulb adequately for one reason or another. In a very rare instance, the examination has to be performed under general anaesthesia immediately prior to surgery. Endotracheal intubation abolishes the risk of regurgitation and allows generous lavage when necessary.

RECOGNITION OF BLEEDING TYPE

A lesion may be actively bleeding at the time of the examination, or may show stigmata of recent haemorrhage [6]. In the absence of evidence of bleeding a lesion may be the presumed cause or an area may be the presumed site of bleeding.

(a) Visible active bleeding at the time of the examination allows unequivocal incrimination as the bleeding source. The bleeding may be oozing or spurting. The percentage of spurters depends upon the endoscopic policy. The figure may be as high as 25% in hospitals which routinely provide emergency endoscopy within a few hours of admission. In the ASGE survey active oozing or pumping bleeding was present in 41.5% of patients during the first 12 hours and dropped to 29.4% of patients examined during the second 12 hours [5]. Usually the percentage of spurting bleeding is less than 10% in the majority of hospitals with a less aggressive approach. It is not uncommon to observe active bleeding in an ulcer or varix or Mallory–Weiss tear which stops and starts during the endoscopic examination.

(b) Stigmata of recent haemorrhage include the presence of an adherent clot which cannot be washed off with a powerful jet of water to demonstrate that it is adherent, the presence of a visible vessel or the presence of an ulcer, whose base is haemorrhagic, either showing a darkened slough or a dark spot at the original site of the bleeding. These stigmata, when present, offer reasonable evidence that such lesions have recently bled. Such stigmata are particularly prevalent in gastric ulcers, duodenal ulcers, Mallory–Weiss tears and oesophageal varices. Such stigmata can disappear rather fast, especially from duodenal ulcers, tears and varices.

(c) If the patient has presented with haematemesis and endoscopy shows only a single lesion, even without any of the stigmata of recent bleeding, it is likely to be the bleeding source. Such a single lesion has to be found in a complete survey of oesophagus, stomach and the first two parts of the duodenum. In practice, it is not uncommon to find gastric or duodenal ulcers with a clean base without blood in the stomach, when such patients have stopped bleeding prior to admission. A single lesion cannot be considered the presumed cause of bleeding when the presentation has been only with melena or if the examination takes place more than 48 hours after the bleeding episode, since acute lesions, such as tears and erosions may already have healed at that time.

(d) If profuse bleeding prevents visualization of the cause of the bleeding, it may only be possible to diagnose a presumed site by excluding bleeding lesions in certain areas, for example bleeding from the bulb in the absence of any lesion in the stomach or oesophagus or massive bleeding in the proximal intestinal tract in the absence of any visible lesion in the oesophagus.

RECOGNITION OF BLEEDING LESIONS

The spectrum of lesions which can be diagnosed endoscopically varies substantially between countries and also according to the nature of the admitting hospital. A global estimate of the relative frequencies of bleeding lesions is summarized in Table 1.1.

Approximately 10–20% of bleeding patients are found to have two or more mucosal lesions such as the combination of duodenal ulcers and acute erosions. In the ASGE study, multiple endoscopic findings were observed in 33.2% of cases [5].

Table 1.1 Range of endoscopically detected bleeding causes

Oesophagus	
Varices	5–20%
Oesophagitis	5–10%
Oesophageal ulcer (Barrett)	<3%
Mallory–Weiss tear	5–15%
Neoplasm, prosthesis, vascular malformation	<5%
Stomach	
Peptic ulcer	15–20%
Erosive haemorrhagic gastritis	10–20%
Neoplasm	<5%
Hiatal hernia	<2%
Vascular malformation	<2%
Duodenum	
Peptic ulcer	20–25%
Stomal (anastomotic ulcer)	1–5%
(Erosive) duodenitis	5–10%

Therefore a complete examination of the whole proximal intestinal tract should always be performed, no matter what is seen *en route*.

(a) The importance of *varices* shows a striking geographical variation, reflecting the prevalence of alcoholic liver damage except for areas with endemic schistosomiasis. Varices are detectable as submucosal swellings, that may run longitudinally in the oesophagus as sinuous cords, or, when very large they have a knotted appearance and even resemble clusters of grapes. They may have a blue or bluish-red colour on endoscopic inspection, but at other times, their colour may be identical to the surrounding mucosa. They are initially maximally prominent near the oesophagogastric junction but may extend into the cardia of the stomach or up to the oesophagus as high as the aortic arch. There is a general relationship between variceal size and likelihood of haemorrhage [7, 8, 9, 10]. Bleeding from gastric mucosal lesions is more frequent in the presence of large gastro-oesophageal varices. Approximately one-third to one-half of the bleeding episodes in cirrhotics are caused by gastritis or other abnormalities. In patients with alcoholic cirrhosis, bleeding from varices and gastric erosions is equally common, but peptic ulceration and Mallory–Weiss tears may also account for up to 20% of bleeding episodes [11, 12]. In patients with non-alcoholic liver disease, a variceal source can be identified in up to 80% of examinations. In the large scale American ASGE survey, the presence of varices was associated in 33.7% with another lesion which was designated as the final cause of bleeding [5]. The diagnosis of variceal haemorrhage is confirmed if active bleeding is identified from a varix, if a varix is seen with a strongly adherent clot or if varices are found as the only lesion in the absence of another potential bleeding site.

(b) Endoscopy has highlighted the importance of oesophagitis, especially in elderly recumbent patients as a cause of bleeding. Massive bleeding from reflux oesophagitis is rather uncommon although occasionally spurting haemorrhage may be observed. Although the presence of blood in the oesophagus already suggests an oesophageal source, one should always try to get an adequate view by removing blood or refluxed gastric contents from the mucosa through irrigation. Bleeding from an already inflamed oesophageal mucosa may be precipitated by prolonged presence of irritant tablets because of defective oesophageal clearance. It is surprising that a prior history of dyspepsia, nocturnal chest pain or sour regurgitation is often lacking.

Overt upper alimentary bleeding is much more often due to a chronic ulceration, usually in a *columnar-lined* oesophagus (*Barrett ulcer*). Such ulcers resemble ordinary chronic gastric ulcers in that they are deep and solitary with a white base and sharply defined edges. In a rare instance such ulcers may penetrate into the aorta causing torrential bleeding. In addition recurrent bleeding from such ulcers is not uncommon.

(c) A wide variation in the incidence of *Mallory–Weiss tears* is apparent in the reported series accounting for between 5–15% of all acute upper alimentary bleeding episodes. One or occasionally more longitudinal mucosal tears are visible at the level of the cardia, at or just below the squamocolumnar mucosal junction. In this region, the submucosa contains a plexus of thin-walled vessels which constitute the source of bleeding. A small sliding hiatal hernia can be found in the majority of patients. Bleeding usually occurs when the cardia is in the thorax, at which time any violent diaphragmatic contraction with increase of intra-abdominal pressure will subject this cardiac region to a very high pressure gradient across its wall [13]. The endoscopist should first carefully inspect the cardia from the oesophageal side ahead of the instrument, looking for signs of bleeding or adherent clot. The instrument is then passed through the cardia and put through a U-turn to examine the gastric side of the cardia which is the more common side for tears to occur. In the ASGE series, 24 tears were oesophageal, 100 were junctional and 46 were gastric [5]. It is essential to decide whether a Mallory–Weiss tear is present before proceeding to the examination of the remainder of the stomach and duodenum since tearing can occur during endoscopy if severe retching occurs. Gentle irrigation of a tear will usually clear sufficient blood to reveal the fissured lesion with gaping edges. After 2–3 days the tear is converted into a linear ulcer with a grayish base which is usually completely healed after 7–10 days. The diagnosis of a Mallory–Weiss tear is suggested by the sequens of emesis followed by haematemesis but more than 50% of patients give no history of retching or vomiting [14]. Many but not all the patients have a heavy intake of alcohol [15].

(d) *Oesophageal neoplasms* are an uncommon cause of bleeding. After palliative intubation with a prosthesis, pressure necrosis may occur which occasionally causes haemorrhage. Exceptionally such pressure necrosis may even extend into the aorta causing torrential bleeding. This may however also occur by direct invasion by a squamous carcinoma in an unintubated patient. Rendu–Osler telangiectases may occasionally occur in the oesophageal mucosa.

(e) *Peptic ulceration* of the *gastric* or *duodenal mucosa* is the most common cause of bleeding. A duodenal ulcer is the source of bleeding in about one-third and a gastric ulcer in about one-fifth of the patients admitted with alimentary bleeding. Stomal ulceration is less common although bleeding is reported to occur in about a third of patients with a recurrent stomal ulcer. Acute ulcers which bleed are usually flat and may involve small arteries and veins before they have had time to undergo thrombotic obliteration. Diffuse slow bleeding is more common in such an oedematous inflamed lesion. More intense ozzing may result if the area is particularly vascular and acutely inflamed. Even whilst healing vessels may rupture and then commonly project, nipple-like, from the centre.

In chronic ulcers with endarteritis obliterans changes in arteries and thrombotic changes in veins, usually a saccular aneurysm develops prior to rupture, causing a breach in the vessel wall. This causes profuse haemorrhage from a sideways-ruptured major artery in the base of a penetrating ulcer. The most common sites for bleeding ulcers are the lesser curvature or posterior wall of the stomach and the posterior wall of the duodenum. After a slightly greater tendency to haemorrhage in the first years, it appears that the incidence of bleeding in peptic ulcer patients then remains more or less constant at about 5% per annum up to ten years, when there might be some reduction. The longer the duration of ulcer disease, the greater the chance that the patient will have bled. Apart from a substantial number of bleeding duodenal ulcers in younger men, the rates of haemorrhage in both types of ulcer are at least five times higher over the age of 50. The chance of further haemorrhage appears to be greater in patients who have already bled [16]. An ulcer which begins later in life, either gastric or duodenal, is more prone to bleed than a longstanding ulcer present before the age of 30. Painless haemorrhage may occur, somewhat more in gastric than in duodenal ulcer patients.

In the ASGE study 41% of patients with a prior history of ulcer had a different source for their bleeding episode [5], confirming the relatively poor predictive value of prior history of a specific disease on current endoscopic findings.

(f) Most large series report an incidence of approximately 10–20% for *erosive haemorrhagic gastritis* as the cause of the bleeding. In the recent ASGE study, gastric erosions were the most commonly observed bleeding lesion. The term 'haemorrhagic gastritis' simply defines the background gastric mucosal lesion upon which are sometimes superimposed acute superficial erosions and ulcers. Erosions are by definition shallow, usually less than 5 mm in diameter and oval or circular in shape. Their edges are sharply defined, raised and congested and their base grayish yellow. They have a tendency to be present in chains or clusters, more commonly in the antrum. It has been said that the reliability of detecting erosions could be considerably improved if dye-scattering techniques are used to define the existence of erosions [17]. Since acute erosions (epithelial necrosis superficial to the muscularis mucosae) may progress to true ulcers extending into the submucosa, there seems little point in attempting to differentiate these because they are pathogenetically and clinically similar. Extension of the ulcerative process into the submucosal layer where major blood vessels are present is more likely to be associated with major haemorrhage. The intervening mucosa around erosions is often congested and oedematous and coated by large amounts of mucus.

There may be well-defined petechial haemorrhages, larger zones of confluent mucosal or submucosal bleeding areas together with free bleeding from the surface of the erosions. Care must be taken to confirm that a demonstrable lesion is in fact bleeding and not just smeared with fresh blood. Endoscopy must be carried out quickly to make this diagnosis as erosions may heal rapidly. Endoscopy within 12 hours of a bleeding episode has indicated rates of incidence as high as 33% [18] and even 68% [19]. Bleeding from acute erosions is often from multiple vessels or from the end of a single artery. Erosions occur in many conditions associated with stress such as severe trauma, burns (Curling's ulcer), head injury (Cushing's ulcer), cerebrovascular accidents, major infection, respiratory failure and many metabolic derangements which have been proposed as precipitating factors. Most commonly, acute stress ulceration begins as multiple shallow ulcerations which are located in the fundic region of the stomach. Submucosal scarring is completely absent which is consistent with the fact that these lesions occur within minutes to hours of an acute episode of trauma or other serious illness. Initially such erosions are multiple, shallow and red based. Gradually they become deeper and black based with swelling at the margin. Gradually they may spread to involve the entire body of the stomach. Early gastroscopic studies have provided clear evidence that erosive damage can also follow ingestion of salicylate and other antiphlogistic drugs.

Finally many patients admitted to hospital with erosive bleeding do not have a definable cause or do not have any of the mentioned precipitating factors (idiopathic erosions).

(g) *Gastric neoplasm, vascular malformation* or *hiatal hernia* is a less common cause of upper intestinal bleeding. Bulky necrotic ulcerating tumors usually create no diagnostic difficulty. Flat, superficial ulcers causing bleeding may look benign although, in reality are caused by early gastric cancer. Biopsies which are usually obtained after the arrest of bleeding are mandatory to detect the true nature of such lesions. Endoscopists should be aware that upper intestinal bleeding as a presenting symptom of an early gastric cancer is by no means an exception.

Telangiectases (Rendu–Osler–Weber disease) usually occur in gastric mucosa and are liable to bleed. Such vascular lesions were present in the ASGE survey in 0.5% of cases [5]. Usually there is no blood in the stomach or at the most slight oozing from these vascular abnormalities may be observed.

Apart from associated oesophagitis, hiatal hernia may cause alimentary bleeding from mucosal trauma at the diaphragmatic level. Trauma at the hiatal level, usually due to a tight hiatus, causes a chronic gastric 'riding' ulcer which develops astride the hiatus. This may be the cause of massive bleeding. In addition erosions may occur in the hiatal sack, more often in association with para-oesophageal than with sliding hernias.

(h) *Erosive duodenitis*, usually characterized by diffuse inflammation of the mucosa in the duodenal bulb, often with scattered erosions without a detectable ulcer crater is not uncommon. Antispasmodic medication may be helpful when there is severe spasm hindering adequate duodenal inspection. In the ASGE survey erosive duodenitis was present in 9% of cases [5]. To what extent drug intake or alcohol abuse is responsible for such lesions is unknown at present.

DIAGNOSTIC ACCURACY AND PROGNOSTIC IMPLICATIONS

The diagnostic accuracy is dependent upon the skill and experience of the endoscopist and the adequacy of facilities, equipment and supporting personnel. The importance cannot be overstressed for adequate patient preparation, patience and the need on occasion to wash out the stomach and repeat the procedure. If the procedure is incomplete, the patient is best re-endoscoped 12–24 hours later.

Although performing upper gastrointestinal panendoscopy is difficult in the bleeding patient, the well-trained endoscopist can in the majority of circumstances locate the bleeding lesion and, in those cases in which there is more than one potentially bleeding lesion, identify the one responsible for most of the bleeding. Most authors of large series claim a diagnostic accuracy of 80–95% [2, 18, 20–23]. Some failures are inevitable due to profuse bleeding or poor patient tolerance.

The information gathered during emergency endoscopy provides important prognostic information. In general, varices are more likely to rebleed than ulcers and ulcers more likely to rebleed than erosions or hiatal hernia [24]. Patients with active (oozing or spurting) bleeding or with stigmata of recent haemorrhage in gastric or duodenal ulcers (protruding visible vessels) are far more likely to rebleed and require emergency surgery than those whose bases are clean or show only one small central spot [5, 6, 21, 25, 26]. Morgan *et al.* [27] found six factors to connote a poor prognosis. These comprised: age over 60, a past medical history of cardiac, respiratory, hepatic or renal disease, absence of recent alcohol intake or absence of recent medication ingestion, endoscopic evidence of an ulcer or cancer and the presence of congestive heart failure noted upon admission. A patient with three or more of these factors had an increased risk of rebleeding and mortality. The recently published large scale American survey of bleeding patients largely substantiated these findings. According to Gilbert *et al.* [5], increased mortality was associated with increased age, underlying disease, including cardiopulmonary and malignant illness, liver disease, absence of recent salicytate intake, and severity of bleeding. In addition, the endoscopic observation of an oozing or pumping lesion was a similarly useful predictor of outcome [3, 5].

COMPLICATIONS OF EMERGENCY ENDOSCOPY

Any endoscopic procedure in a seriously ill patient is potentially hazardous although the precise risks in acute bleeding are insufficiently documented. Emergency endoscopy is generally considered to be more hazardous than routine endoscopy [2, 5, 28–31]. Critics of emergency endoscopy argue that the stomach often contains blood which can be aspirated into the lungs during the procedure and that instrumentation may aggravate the bleeding by dislodging haemostatic clots from the surface of a bleeding lesion. The possibility of restarting bleeding by active removal of a clot from a base of an ulcer or other lesion cannot be denied although aggravation of bleeding in other circumstances is presumably very rare.

The overall complication rate in the ASGE survey on upper gastrointestinal bleeding was 0.9% [2]. The major complications were perforation, aspiration pneumonia and reactivation of haemorrhage. The mortality attributable to endoscopy was estimated as 0.13% of patients [5]. Other endoscopic series confined to patients with upper gastrointestinal bleeding have shown associated complication rates ranging from 0.7% to as high as 8% [1, 18, 32, 33]. The last high figure of 8% was obtained in severely ill patients with bleeding, managed in intensive care units.

To some extent the possibility of complications can perhaps be reduced. Emergency endoscopy requires more skill and clinical judgement and should therefore not be dedicated to physicians at an early stage of training. The possibility of pulmonary aspiration can probably be reduced by avoiding heavy sedation. Less experienced endoscopists tend to use more sedation, which increases the risk of bronchopulmonary aspiration and may aggravate any cardiorespiratory or hepatic insufficiency [34]. Endoscopy should not be performed in patients with uncontrollable agitation and in those with torrential bleeding. Because bleeding can be precipitated or aggravated during attempts to clean an ulcer base, this should probably only be performed when possibilities for local haemostasis are available.

POTENTIAL VALUE OF EMERGENCY ENDOSCOPY

There is more or less general agreement about several beneficial aspects of emergency endoscopy although the impact is difficult to quantify.

A major benefit of emergency endoscopy is certainly the insurance that most bleeding patients are seen, fairly rapidly by an experienced gastroenterologist or, in other circumstances, the creation of a combined medical–surgical approach in which patients are cared for by the same personnel, familiar with all aspects of upper gastrointestinal bleeding.

In addition precise determination of the location and type of bleeding may be of particular value to the surgeon. Preoperative knowledge of the exact nature and site of bleeding influences the placement of the appropriate incision line, increases the speed and the smoothness with which the procedure can be accomplished and avoids the need for unnecessary intraoperative manoeuvres which might increase morbidity and mortality.

Furthermore one of the major benefits of precise endoscopic diagnosis is avoidance of an inappropriate operation e.g. in patients bleeding from oesophageal varices or diffuse erosive gastritis. Also the physician is helped with a specific diagnosis. He can avoid the use of potentially harmful techniques, or he may discontinue ineffective therapies, or he may identify the lesions whose cause may be affected by therapy. Counselling of the patient or the family may be more rational and a better estimate of long-term prognosis may be possible.

Since endoscopy is considered in general to be the most accurate diagnostic procedure the question can be raised whether early endoscopy is worth while and whether emergency endoscopy does improve the outcome of the patient [35–37]. Several controlled investigations were undertaken to evaluate the effect of early endoscopy on outcome in patients with upper gastrointestinal tract haemorrhage (Table 1.2). In these studies which included several hundreds of patients, neither the mortality rate, the number of transfusions, the need for surgery nor the duration of hospitalization were improved by emergency endoscopy despite more accurate indentification of the site of bleeding. Thus despite more rapid and more accurate diagnosis by early endoscopy the outcome of therapy was not improved. Major criticisms can be raised with respect to several of these studies.

In the Nottingham trial [40, 41], some patients underwent endoscopy more than 24 hours after admission which may have reduced the surprisingly low diagnostic accuracy of endoscopy. Furthermore, there was no method of

Table 1.2 Impact of emergency endoscopy upon patient survival

Study design*	No. of patients	Endoscopic accuracy (%)	Peptic ulcer (%)	Oesophageal varices (%)	Surgery (%)	Mortality of emergency endoscopy group (%)	Statistically significant from control value (p)
Allan and Dykes, 1974 [38]	EE+Ro vs. SE+Ro	100		19	1		8	neg
Sandlow et al., 1974 [39]	EE+Ro vs. E+Ro after 1 week	150	67	46	5	7	7.5	neg
Dronfield et al., 1977 [40, 41]	EE vs. Ro	1037	73	48	1	18	8.4	neg
Graham, 1980 [42]	EE vs. 4 d delayed EE results	95		48	20		11	neg
Peterson et al., 1981† [43]	EE+Ro vs. Ro+SE	206	84	40	20	13	11	neg

* E endoscopy; EE emergency endoscopy; SE selective endoscopy; Ro upper gastrointestinal radiology.
† Patients were selected in whom bleeding had ceased within 6 h of hospital admission.

standardizing therapy for patients in the endoscopy versus radiology group and patients were not followed up after discharge in order to determine any long range outcome differences.

Peterson's study [43] was based on the observation that the great majority of patients stabilize with conservative medical management and that bleeding does not recur in the majority of patients. In that study, patients were randomly allocated to early endoscopy when their condition had stabilized within six hours of treatment with an empiric antacid regimen. Stabilization was said to have occurred when there was only minimal active bleeding with gastric lavage. In 6% continued bleeding occurred which required urgent endoscopy and surgery.

Making a diagnosis in Peterson's study did not influence outcome which is not at all surprising since therapy was not affected. Why should endoscopy disclose a significant difference when the result of endoscopy did not dictate therapy? Another major criticism against Peterson's study is the standardized antacid treatment for all lesions irrespective their nature. Antacid therapy is certainly not the most appropriate treatment for patients with bleeding oesophageal varices. Note that oesophageal varices accounted for 33% of recurrent bleeding.

The main problem is that an accurate diagnosis by whatever means is not in itself beneficial. If more accurate diagnosis does not lead to better patient management, surely the management must be wrong or inefficient. In his editorial Conn [44] also states that one must be careful not to fault the diagnostic technique for the faults of the therapy. The diagnostic value of emergency endoscopy in patients with, for example, variceal haemorrhage can be demonstrated only in controlled investigations in which early correct diagnosis is linked to early definitive therapy such as perhaps sclerotherapy.

Although it seems likely that improvement in diagnostic precision will ultimately reduce mortality and morbidity resulting from surgery, this has not yet been clearly demonstrated. Very probably this situation results from our inability to identify specific subsets of patients with upper gastrointestinal haemorrhage who would benefit from early and specific diagnosis. In addition definite and effective therapy for identifiable lesions is not yet fully developed.

The current lack of effect on overall mortality suggests that the major task for the near future is to use the diagnostic information gained by endoscopy as a stimulus for further vigorous investigations of different and newer therapies.

CONCLUSIONS

Emergency endoscopy is now a routine procedure. Early diagnosis is considered useful. Those accustomed to using early endoscopy would now find it difficult and uncomfortable to manage the patients without it. A firm diagnosis is useful in avoiding inappropriate management. Surgeons believe that the task is made easier by previous diagnosis, particularly when the source of bleeding lies in the chest. Early diagnosis is also believed to allow the selection of high risk patients who can then be treated appropriately. It is beyond doubt that the full impact of improved diagnostic accuracy will only be discernible when the diagnostic information is followed by more appropriate therapeutic decisions. Emergency endoscopy may prove to be a major advance when better control of variceal bleeding through endoscopic sclerotherapy is obtained, when better control of oozing or spurting haemorrhage by local haemostatic devices is possible and when better selection of patients for rapid elective surgery in order to prevent rebleeding is recognized and adopted on a large scale. It is to be expected that in the future morbidity and mortality of acute bleeding will be increasingly related to underlying diseases, which will be difficult to improve no matter which diagnostic principle is used.

REFERENCES

1. Allen, R. and Dykes, P. A. (1976) A study of the factors influencing mortality rates from gastrointestinal hemorrhage. *Q. J. Med.* **45**, 533–50.
2. Silverstein, F. E., Gilbert, D. A., Tedesco, F. J., Buenger, N. K. and Persing, J. (1981a) The national ASGE survey on upper gastrointestinal bleeding. I Study design and baseline data. *Gastrointest. Endosc.* **27**, 73–9.
3. Silverstein, F. E., Gilbert, D. A., Tedesco, F. J., Buenger, N. K. and Persing, J. (1981b) The national ASGE survey on upper gastrointestinal bleeding. II Clinical prognostic factors. *Gastrointest. Endosc.* **27**, 80–93.
4. Forrest, J. A. H., Finlayson, N. D. C. and Shearman, D. J. C. (1974) Endoscopy in gastrointestinal bleeding. *Lancet*, **ii**, 394–7.
5. Gilbert, D. A., Silverstein, F. E., Tedesco, F. J., Buenger, N. K. and Persing, J. (1981) The National ASGE survey on upper gastrointestinal bleeding. III Endoscopy in upper gastrointestinal bleeding. *Gastrointest. Endosc.*, **27**, 94–102.
6. Foster, D. N., Miloszewski, K. J. A. and Losowsky, M. S. (1977) Stigmata of recent haemorrhage in diagnosis and prognosis of upper gastrointestinal bleeding. *Br. Med. J.*, I, 1173–7.
7. Baker, L. A., Smith, C. and Lieberman, G. (1959) The natural history of esophageal varices. A study of 115 cirrhotic patients in whom varices were diagnosed prior to bleeding. *Am. J. Med.*, **26**, 228–37.
8. Dagradi, A. E. (1972) The natural history of esophageal varices in patients with alcoholic liver cirrhosis: an endoscopic and clinical study. *Am. J. Gastroenterol.*, **57**, 520–40.
9. Dagradi, A. E., Mehler, R., Tan, D. T. D. and Stempien, S. J. (1970) Sources of upper gastrointestinal bleeding in patients with liver cirrhosis and large esophagogastric varices. *Am. J. Gastroenterol.*, **54**, 458–63.
10. Palmer, E. D. and Brick, I. B. (1956) Correlation between the severity of esophageal varices in portal cirrhosis and their propensity toward hemorrhage. *Gastroenterology*, **30**, 85–90.
11. McCray, R. C., Martin, F., Amir-Ahmadi, H., Sheahan, D. G. and Zamcheck, N. (1969) Erroneous diagnosis of hemorrhage from esophageal varices. *Am. J. Dig. Dis.*, **14**, 755–60.
12. Waldram, R., Davis, M., Nunnerly, H. and Williams, R. (1974) Emergency endoscopy after gastrointestinal haemorrhage in 50 patients with portal hypertension. *Br. Med. J.*, 4, 94–6.
13. Atkinson, M., Bottrill, M. B. and Edwards, A. T. (1961) Mucosal tears at the oesophagogastric junction (Mallory–Weiss syndrome). *Gut*, **2**, 1–11.

14. Foster, D. N., Miloszewski, K. and Losowsky, M. S. (1976) Diagnosis of Mallory–Weiss lesions – a common cause of upper gastrointestinal bleeding. *Lancet*, **ii**, 483–5.
15. Mallory, E. K. and Weiss, S. (1929) Haemorrhages from lacerations of the cardiac orifice of the stomach due to vomiting. *Am. J. Med. Sci.*, **178**, 506–75.
16. Jordan, S. M. and Kiefer, E. D. (1934) Complications of peptic ulcer: their prognostic significance. *JAMA*, **103**, 2004–7.
17. Kohli, Y., Nakajima, M., Ida, K. and Kawai, K. (1974) Minute endoscopical findings of duodenal mucosa using the dye scattering method. *Endoscopy*, **6**, 1–6.
18. Cotton, P. B., Rosenberg, M. T., Waldram, R. P. L. and Axon, A. T. R. (1973) Early endoscopy of oesophagus, stomach and duodenal bulb in patients with haematemesis and melaena. *Br. Med. J.*, **2**, 505–9.
19. Sugawa, C., Werner, M. H., Hayes, D. F., Lucas, C. E. and Walt, A. J. (1973) Early endoscopy. A guide to therapy for acute hemorrhage in the upper gastrointestinal tract. *Arch. Surg.*, **107**, 133–7.
20. Iglesias, M. C., Dourdourekas, D. and Adomavicius, J. (1979) Prompt endoscopic diagnosis of upper gastrointestinal haemorrhage: its value for specific diagnosis and management. *Ann. Surg.*, **189**, 90–5.
21. Laurence, B. H., Vallon, A. G., Cotton, P. B., Miro, J. R. A. *et al.* (1980) Endoscopic laser photocoagulation for bleeding peptic ulcers. *Lancet*, **i**, 124–5.
22. Meuwissen, S. G. M., Pape, K. S. S. B., van Tetering, J. P. B. and Tytgat, G. N. (1975) 'Acute' endoscopie bij bloedingen uit het bovengedeelte van de tractus digestivus. *Ned Tijdschr Geneesk*, **119**, 52–6.
23. Thomas, G. E., Cotton, P. B., Clark, C. G. and Boulos, P. B. (1978) Survey of management of acute upper gastrointestinal haemorrhage. *J. R. Soc. Med.*, **73**, 90–5.
24. Jones, P. F., Johnston, S. J. and McEwan, A. R. (1973) Further haemorrhage after admission to hospital for gastrointestinal haemorrhage. *Br. Med. J.*, **3**, 660–4.
25. Griffiths, W. J., Neumann, D. A. and Welsh, J. D. (1979) The visible vessel as an indicator of uncontrolled or recurrent gastrointestinal haemorrhage. *New Engl. J. Med.*, **300**, 1411–13.
26. Salmon, P. R. (1974) *Fibreoptic Endoscopy*, Pitman Medical, London.
27. Morgan, A. G., McAdam, W. A. F., Walmisley, G. L., Jessop, A. *et al.* (1977) Clinical findings, early endoscopy, and multivariate analysis in patients bleeding from the upper gastrointestinal tract. *Br. Med. J.*, **2**, 237–40.
28. Davis, R. E. and Graham, D. Y. (1979) Endoscopic complications. *Gastrointest. Endosc.*, **25**, 146–9.
29. Schiller, K. F. R. and Prout, B. J. (1976) in *Topics in Gastrointestinal Endoscopy*, (eds K. F. R. Schiller and P. R. Salmon), Heinemann, London, pp. 147–65.
30. Stadelmann, O., Karp, E. and Meiderers, S. E. (1974) in *Advances in Endoscopy*, (ed. R. Ottenjann), F. K. Schattauer Verlag, Stuttgart, pp. 1–5.
31. Katon, R. M. (1981) Complications of upper gastrointestinal endoscopy in the gastrointestinal bleeder. *Dig. Dis. Sci.*, **26**, 470.
32. Palmer, E. D. (1969) The vigorous diagnostic approach to upper gastrointestinal tract hemorrhage. *JAMA*, **207**, 1477–80.
33. Paul, F. and Huchzermeyer, H. (1980) in *Abstracts of the IVth European Congress of Gastrointestinal Endoscopy*, Georg Thieme Verlag, Stuttgart, p. 103.
34. Schiller, K. F. R. and Cotton, P. B. (1978) Acute upper gastrointestinal haemorrhage. *Clin. Gastroenterol.*, **7**, 595–604.
35. Eastwood, G. L. (1977) Does early endoscopy benefit the patient with active upper gastrointestinal bleeding? *Gastroenterology*, **72**, 737–9.
36. Eastwood, G. L. (1981) Does the patient with upper gastrointestinal bleeding benefit from endoscopy? *Dig. Dis. Sci.*, **26**, 225.
37. Winans, C. S. (1977) Emergency upper gastrointestinal endoscopy: does haste make waste? *Dig. Dis.*, **22**, 536–40.

38. Allan, R. and Dykes, P. A. (1974) A comparison of routine and selective endoscopy in the management of acute gastrointestinal hemorrhage. *Gastrointest. Endosc.*, **20**, 154–5.

39. Sandlow, L. J., Becker, G. H., Spellberg, M. A., Allen, H. A. *et al.* (1974) A prospective randomized study of the management of upper gastrointestinal hemorrhage. *Am. J. Gastroenterol.*, **61**, 282–9.

40. Dronfield, M. W., Ferguson, R., McIllmurray, M. B., Atkinson, M. and Langman, M. J. S. (1977) A prospective randomised study of endoscopy and radiology in acute upper gastrointestinal tract bleeding. *Lancet*, **i**, 1167–8.

41. Dronfield, M. W., Langman, M. J. S., Atkinson, M. *et al.* (1982) Outcome of endoscopy and barium radiography for acute upper gastrointestinal bleeding: controlled trial in 1037 patients. *Br. Med. J.*, **284**, 545.

42. Graham, D. Y. (1980) Limited value of early endoscopy in the management of acute upper gastrointestinal bleeding: prospective controlled trial. *Am. J. Surg.*, **140**, 284–90.

43. Peterson, W. L., Barnett, C. C., Smith, H. J., Allen, M. H. and Corbett, D. B. (1981) Routine early endoscopy in upper gastrointestinal tract bleeding. A randomized controlled trial. *New Engl. J. Med.*, **304**, 925–9.

44. Conn, H. O. (1981) To scope or not to scope. *New Engl. J. Med.*, **304**, 967–9.

2

Endoscopic electrocoagulation

P. FRÜHMORGEN, W. MATEK and L. DEMLING

Several methods used to control gastrointestinal haemorrhage by endoscopy are discussed in this chapter and some of them are used experimentally or clinically although no prospective and randomized studies have been made [1, 2, 3, 4].

To obtain objective and comparable results we treated standardized bleeding stomach ulcers [5] gastrotomized and heparinized dogs using the different methods of haemo-clip, haemostyptics, lasers (Argon and Neodymium Yttrium Aluminium Garnet (Nd YAG), conventional electrocoagulation and modifications of electrocoagulation.

The results indicated very clearly that only photocoagulation by lasers and electrocoagulation are highly effective in controlling standardized bleeding [6].

Disadvantages of the simple electrocoagulation, which is cheaper than lasers and more mobile, are well known (Table 2.1). Therefore we developed a modified electrocoagulation with the advantages of laser coagulation excluding the disadvantages of photocoagulation (eg. expensive and immovable).

Table 2.1 Well-known disadvantages of the simple electrocoagulation

---

1) Bad visibility
2) Adhesion of the electrode to the spot to be coagulated
3) Adhesion of carbonized material at the electrode
4) Secondary enlargement of the coagulated area
5) High risk of perforation

MATERIALS AND METHODS

The high-frequency current (Electrotom 170 RF machine from Martin, Germany, 10-step power switch, maximum output of 170 watts), a so-called coagulation current, was used for coagulation with modified monopolar electrodes. We injected or insufflated different fluids or gas (Table 2.2) through five small holes in the tip of the electrode. A spring mechanism guarantees that the electrode is pressed against the tissue with nearly constant force. With the first step of a 2-step switch controlled by the foot of the endoscopist, the bleeding site was blown or rinsed free of the blood covering it using gas or the mentioned fluids, also used during electrocoagulation with the second step of the switch. The liquids were injected at a rate of 20–40 ml min^{-1}.

The time and output levels of our coagulation system required to stop the standardized bleeding and the macroscopic and microscopic tissue changes in acute and chronic animal experiments were noted in order to narrow down the effectivity and therapeutic range [7, 8]. After we finished our animal experiments we started to treat patients with the best of all tested methods.

Table 2.2 Tested modifications of electrocoagulation

Electrocoagulation with:
1) Simultaneous insufflation of gas (CO_2)
2) Simultaneous instillation of water
3) Simultaneous instillation of physiological salt solution
4) 'Ionized liquid' (without contact of the electrode to the spot to be coagulated)
5) Simultaneous instillation of haemostyptics

RESULTS

Acute experiments [8]

Using electrocoagulation with simultaneous *insufflation of gas* (CO_2) output levels of 8, 9 and 10 were necessary in order to control bleeding. The visibility during simultaneous gas insufflation was good but adherence of coagulated material to the electrode was not completely eliminated. The therapeutic range of the treatment time was limited to about 15 seconds in the stomach. Of 19 bleedings all were controlled within the limits of the therapeutic range. But the depth of penetration extended in seven cases to the outer layers of the muscularis propria.

Electrocoagulation with simultaneous *instillation of distilled water* (EHT probe) using output level 6, which was sufficient to control all of 20 bleedings, demonstrated very good visibility at the source of the bleeding, showed no adhesion to the electrode and no carbonization of the tissue. The middle and outer layers of the muscularis propria of the stomach were histologically never reached by coagulation, even using coagulation times up to 180 seconds. For this reason using output level 6 no time limit was needed and all 20 bleedings were arrested within the therapeutic range without perforations.

The result of *instillation of physiological saline solution* was identical to those found with simultaneous instillation of water. Only macroscopically there was a distinct hyperaemia surrounding the coagulated ulcer. Using *concentrated saline solution* arrest of bleeding was achieved in only two of 20 cases by level 6, resulting in a large superficial coagulation area.

Simultaneous *instillation of hydrogen peroxide* (H_2O_2) led to such extreme foaming that the bleeding site to be coagulated was no longer clearly visible (Table 2.3).

Chronic experiments [8]

Prior to clinical application of the best of our tested methods we investigated the process of healing of the coagulated bleeding ulcers using the so-called EHT probe.

Fifty bleeding ulcers were successfully arrested by EHT-coagulation; with the exception of two cases all ulcers healed without complications. Even when the output power was about 30% higher than the minimum power necessary for haemostatic coagulation, no complications were observed. Only using output level 8 with an additional postbleeding-arrest coagulation in excess of ten seconds, two primary perforations in two out of 12 cases were produced. With additional coagulation (at power setting 6 output for 20 seconds eight cases, at power setting 7 for ten seconds six cases) no perforations were observed (Table 2.4). Thus, the therapeutic range seems to be adequately large.

Clinical results

Within the area of emergency endoscopy, the newly developed EHT probe has proved an effective instrument for haemostasis. We have treated 32 patients who presented with active gastrointestinal bleeding. Primary haemostasis was completely successful in 30 cases, and only partially successful in two. Four patients with recurrent bleeds were subjected to surgery (Table 2.5). As had been the case in the animal experiments, owing to the simultaneous instillation of water, in none of the acute gastrointestinal bleeds did the probe adhere to the site of bleeding, or was contaminated by coagulation or charred material. We employed purely coagulation current only. Setting 6 of our coagulation unit (Martin RF 170), which is the smallest effective experimental coagulation setting, proved to be adequate for stopping even arterial bleeding. In the rebleeds, we dispensed with a renewed coagulation in the initial phase of the method, and opted for a surgical procedure. No perforations were observed, and the mortality rate of the method was zero.

DISCUSSION

Acute gastrointestinal bleeding represents an extremely difficult and frequently dramatic problem for operative endoscopy. A solution to this problem through the use of electrocoagulation was sought very early on. In their basic work in this field,

Table 2.3 Electrocoagulation of standardized bleeding

Modification of electro-coagulation (acute experiment dog-stomach)	Visibility	Adhesion of the electrode to the spot to be coagulated	Adhesion of carbonized material to the electrode	Bleedings/ staunched bleedings	Used level of the electrotom	Outer muscularis propria?
Insufflation of gas (CO_2)	good	yes	yes	19/19	8–10	yes ($\times 7$)
Instillation of water	good	no	no	20/20	6	no
Instillation of physiological NaCl-solution	good	no	no	20/20	6	no
'Ionized' liquid	good	no	no	20/2	(6)	no (fibrin)
Instillation of H_2O_2 (haemostyptic)	not good	no	no	5/5	6	no

Table 2.4 EHT probe (chronic experiment, dog-stomach)

Level of coagulation	6	6	7	8
Additional coagulation after cessation of bleeding	0	20	10	10 (s)
Distal point of the scar in:				
Submucosa	21	—	—	3
Muscularis propria (inner part)	3	5	6	5
Muscularis propria (outer part) or seroa	—	3	—	2
Primary perforation	—	—	—	2
Secondary perforation	—	—	—	—
Number of bleedings	24	8	6	12

Table 2.5 Haemostasis with the EHT probe

Nature and localization of the lesion	N	Primary haemostasis successful	Rebleeds
Oesophageal ulcer	2	2	—
Mallory–Weiss syndrome	5	5	1
Gastric ulcer	12	10	1
Duodenal ulcer	3	3	1
Gastric erosion	1	1	—
Gastric carcinoma (after snare biopsy)	1	1	1
Gastric haemangioma	3	3	—
Bleeding after polypectomy			
in the colon	4	4	—
in the stomach	1	1	—
Total	32	30	4

Koch et al. [9] and Pesh et al. [10] found the therapeutic range of electrocoagulation in intact mucous membranes to be very small. Secondary changes with the danger of subsequent perforation reduced the therapeutic range even further. Other working groups have since confirmed their findings [11, 12, 13]. For this reason, endoscopic electrocoagulation as a method of controlling bleeding has hitherto been treated with reserve. It was our aim to check these results, well known in intact mucous membranes, in the case of standardized bleeding in acute and chronic animal experiments.

During coagulation bleeding is a factor that works against perforation: energy which otherwise would penetrate into deeper intestinal layers is carried into the lumen by the flow of blood. A large part of the heat developing in the intestinal wall during coagulation, flows off through the bleeding blood vessel. The cell-damaging energy required for coagulation is thus directed towards the bleeding site. Coagulation of intact mucous membranes produces a wide haemorrhagic border. This is probably due to hyperaemia, intravasal backup of blood and resulting stasis. Secondary enlargement [9, 10] of the coagulated area after several days is probably connected with this local disturbance in bloodflow and the resulting necrobiosis. In the case of bleeding lesions no haemorrhagic border was seen after successful coagulation. It may therefore be concluded that the bleeding itself acts against iatrogenic perforation.

To improve visibility, we insufflated or instilled various agents before and during electrocoagulation. When gas is simultaneously insufflated, a major disadvantage of electrocoagulation already described by Papp *et al.* [11, 12] still remains: the adhesion of coagulated material to the tip of the electrode. For this reason further coagulation is no longer 'calculable'. Covering the electrode with teflon did not help solve this problem [14]. This unpleasant adhesion effect can, however, be completely eliminated by simultaneous instillation of liquids. In this way, the therapeutic range in the cases of bleeding lesions is obviously widened. In contrast to electrocoagulation with simultaneous gas insufflation – whose only advantage over simple coagulation is improved visibility – electrocoagulation with instillation of distilled water (EHT probe) offers distinct advantages (Table 2.6). Other liquids prove to have various technical or medical disadvantages. When saline solutions were used simultaneously, electrocoagulation became more complicated owing to a number of difficult-to-control medical and technical parameters. Concentrated salt solutions lead to additional injury of the mucosa around the bleeding site. Instillation of H_2O_2 reduces visibility at the bleeding site as a result of foam production.

The first results using the EHT probe to control acute gastrointestinal bleeding in patients are encouraging.

Table 2.6 EHT probe

---

1) Optimal visibility at the source of bleeding
2) No adhesion of the probe to the tissue
3) No adhesion of carbonized tissue at the electrode
4) Control of bleeding by pure coagulation
5) Therapeutic range broad enough
6) Lower levels of energy are sufficient to achieve coagulation
7) Safety-range after cessation of bleeding if there was an additional coagulation by mistake

---

SUMMARY

Developing and comparing different types of modified electrocoagulation systems in acute and chronic experiments in dogs electrocoagulation with simultaneous instillation of water (EHT probe) proved the most effective electrocoagulation method to control standardized bleedings. Optimal visibility at the bleeding site, extension of the therapeutic range as well as the avoidance of charring at the bleeding site are its major advantages. Disturbing adhesion of coagulated material on the electrode is also avoided. This method was superior to conventional electrocoagulation, to electrocoagulation with simultaneous insufflation of gas, physiological and concentrated saline solution and haemostyptics.

First applications in 32 patients with acute gastrointestinal bleedings demonstrated that our new EHT probe is a safe, effective, cheap and portable method to control gastrointestinal bleedings. This device might be an real alternative to photocoagulation by lasers.

REFERENCES

1. Demling, L., Frühmorgen, P., Koch, H. and Rösch, W. (1973) in *Operative Endoskopie*, (eds L. Demling, P. Frühmorgen, H. Koch and W. Rösch), Schattauer-Verlag, Stuttgart, pp. 73–7.
2. Frühmorgen, P., Bodem, F., Reidenbach, H-D., Kaduk, B. and Demling, L. (1976) Endoscopic laser coagulation of bleeding gastrointestinal lesions with report of the first therapeutic application in man. *Gastrointest. Endosc.*, **23**, 73–5.
3. Frühmorgen, P., Kaduk, B., Reidenbach, H-D., Bodem, B. *et al.* (1975) Long-term observations in endoscopic laser coagulations in the gastrointestinal tract. *Endoscopy*, **7**, 189–96.
4. Katon, R. M. (1976) Experimental control of gastrointestinal hemorrhagic via endoscopic: a new era dawns. *Gastroenterology*, **70**, 272–7.
5. Matek, W., Frühmorgen, P., Seuberth, K., Kaduk, B. and Demling, L. (1978) Ulcer punch: method and use in animal experiments for the production of standardized lesions and reproducible bleeding in the gastrointestinal tract. *Acta Hepato-Gastroenterol.*, **6**, 450–5.
6. Frühmorgen, P., Matek, W. and Kaduk, B. (1981) Vergleichende Untersuchungen unterschiedlicher Methoden zur gastrointestinalen Blutstillung. *Fortschr. Med.*, **29**, 1140–3.
7. Matek, W., Frühmorgen, P., Kaduk, B., Reidenbach, H-D. *et al.* (1979) Modified electrocoagulation and its possibilities in the control of gastrointestinal bleeding. *Endoscopy*, **4**, 253–8.
8. Matek, W., Frühmorgen, P., Kaduk, B., Reidenbach, H-D. *et al.* (1980) The healing process of experimentally produced bleeding lesions after hemostatic electrocoagulation with simultaneous instillation of water. *Endoscopy*, **12**, 231–6.
9. Koch, H., Pesch, H-J., Bauerle, H., Frühmorgen, P. *et al.* (1972) Erste experimentelle Untersuchungen und klinische Erfahrungen zur Elektrokoagulation blutender Läsionen im oberen Gastrointestinaltrakt. In *Fortschritte der Endoskopie*, vol. 4 (ed. R. Ottenjann), Schattauer-Verlag, Berlin, pp. 69–71.
10. Pesch, H-J., Koch, H. and Classen M. (1973) Experimentelle und histologische Untersuchungen zur Elektrokoagulation blutender Läsionen im oberen Gastro-intestinaltrakt. *Leber Magen Darm*, **3** (4), 172–6.
11. Papp, J. P., Fox, J. M. and Wilks, H. S. (1975) Experimental electrocoagulation of dog gastric mucosa. *Gastrointest. Endosc.*, **22** (1), 27–8.
12. Papp, J. P., Fox, J. M. and Nalbandian, R. M. (1976) Experimental electrocoagulation of dog esophageal and duodenal mucosa. *Gastrointest. Endosc.*, **23**, 27–8.

13. Stadelmann, O., Raschke, E., Müller, R., Löffler, A. and Miederer, S. E. (1973) Endoskopische Elektroresektion und Elektrokoagulation – Voruntersuchungen und erste klinische Erfahrungen. *Fortschritte der Endoskopie*, vol. 4 (ed. R. Ottenjann, Schattauer-Verlag, pp. 63–5.
14. Reidenbach, H-D., Bodem, F., Frühmorgen, P., Schroeder, G. *et al.* (1978) Eine neue Methode zur endoskopischen Hochfrequenzkoagulation von Schleimhautdefekten. *Biomed. Techn. (Berlin)*, **4**, 71.

3

Injection of oesophageal varices

JOHN TERBLANCHE, PHILIP C. BORNMAN and RALPH E. KIRSCH

INTRODUCTION

The combined use of the Sengstaken tube and endoscopic sclerotherapy in the management of the difficult patient with continued bleeding from oesophageal varices has been evaluated prospectively over a five-year period in Cape Town [1]. This presentation summarizes the authors' treatment policy in patients with suspected bleeding varices and compares endoscopic sclerotherapy with other forms of treatment in patients with proven oesophageal variceal bleeding.

INITIAL MANAGEMENT

Patients with massive upper gastrointestinal haemorrhage suspected to be due to bleeding oesophageal varices require admission to hospital, preferably to a centre with a special interest in hepatology. The initial management includes resuscitation with crystalloids plus blood and/or blood components, and careful monitoring, preferably in an intensive care unit.

VASOPRESSIN

Current evidence supports the use of vasopressin, and the Cape Town group believe that it should be administered early, prior to emergency endoscopy, in those patients in whom bleeding oesophageal varices are strongly suspected. Until recently bolus doses of pitressin (20 units in 100 ml of 5% dextrose water) were administered over a 20 minute period and repeated 2–4 hourly, if required.

Recently, pitressin has been administered by continuous intravenous infusion, since this is probably superior to bolus doses [2], and has been shown to be at least as effective as the more complex procedure of intraarterial infusion [3–5]. The current policy is to administer 0.4 units of vasopressin per minute, using an Ivac infusion pump. Two hundred units of vasopressin are diluted to 500 ml in 5% dextrose water and infused at 1 ml min^{-1}. The infusion is commenced when variceal bleeding is suspected and should be continued for 12–24 hours in those patients in whom variceal bleeding is noted to have stopped at the time of emergency endoscopy. Where bleeding is still present at the time of emergency endoscopy, a Sengstaken tube is passed and the vasopressin infusion discontinued.

The synthetic vasopressin analogue, triglycyl lysine vasopressin ('Glypressin'), is under review at present. Its putative advantages are less side effects and ease of administration as bolus doses of 2 mg i.v. six hourly may be as effective as continuous intravenous infusion of vasopressin.

EMERGENCY ENDOSCOPY

Emergency endoscopy is essential to prove that the patient is actually bleeding from oesophageal varices. In a prospective study of emergency endoscopy, one-third of patients in the Cape Town series were shown to be bleeding from a lesion other than their documented oesophageal varices [6]. This has been confirmed in the author's later experience although a greater percentage were actively bleeding from varices at the time of endoscopy (Table 3.1) [1]. Although there are problems with emergency endoscopy in this setting, the authors believe that patients cannot be managed rationally unless the source of bleeding is diagnosed. A confident diagnosis can only be made on emergency endoscopy if a bleeding varix is seen, or if a lesion other than the varices is noted to be bleeding. With massive upper gastrointestinal haemorrhage, vision is often obscured, and the diagnosis of bleeding varices is less secure. It is also essential to perform emergency fibreoptic endoscopy in patients who are readmitted with a suspected variceal bleed after a proven previous variceal bleed. In seven of 27 (26%) subsequent admissions in patients who had originally bled from varices, they were found to be bleeding from a lesion other than their varices [1].

Despite the difficulties, emergency endoscopy separates patients into four groups. The first group do not have varices but have another bleeding lesion. This lesion should be treated on merits. The other three categories include patients who have oesophageal varices on endoscopy (Table 3.1). One group will have varices with active variceal bleeding. The next will have varices in whom the diagnosis of variceal bleeding which has stopped is made. In this setting the diagnosis is based on exclusion of other causes of bleeding in a patient with varices with or without a local blood clot on a varix. Finally, there is the group of patients with varices who have another diagnosed lesion which is actively bleeding.

Patients with varices and another lesion as the source of bleeding are treated on

Table 3.1 Varices on emergency endoscopy: five-year study [1]

Source of bleeding	No. of patients
Active variceal bleeding	71
Variceal bleeding: stopped	33
Varices plus another bleeding lesion	39
Total patients with varices	143

merits. Patients with varices which have stopped bleeding require no further treatment other than continued intravenous pitressin unless they bleed again during that admission. Under these circumstances a Sengstaken tube is passed and they are subjected to injection sclerotherapy. Patients with active variceal bleeding require further definitive measures to stop bleeding. The Cape Town treatment with initial Sengstaken tube tamponade and subsequent injection sclerotherapy is presented below.

SENGSTAKEN TUBE TAMPONADE

Despite the views expressed by Conn that the Sengstaken tube is a potentially dangerous instrument [7, 8], a correctly sited and managed Sengstaken tube will temporarily stop acute variceal bleeding in most patients [1, 9, 10, 11]. It is only dangerous if used without skill. Many of the reported failures are probably due to faulty technique in the hands of inexperienced junior staff. If the patient continues to bleed after the Sengstaken tube has been placed, this indicates either that the tube is incorrectly sited or that the patient is bleeding from another source. The tube should be repositioned and if bleeding continues, repeat emergency endoscopy will usually reveal the other site of bleeding. Although the Sengstaken tube will control bleeding while *in situ*, the rebleed rate on removal of the tube is high. In Cape Town series 60% rebled after removal of the tube [6]. Thus Sengstaken balloon tube tamponade is currently used as a preliminary to more definitive treatment aimed at preventing recurrent bleeding.

The technique of Sengstaken balloon tube tamponade has been detailed elsewhere [12]. The Boyce modification with a fourth oesophageal lumen is preferred [13]. Prior to use the balloons are tested. With the balloons fully deflated and the tube well lubricated, it is passed by the endoscopist at the time of the emergency endoscopy whenever continued variceal bleeding is diagnosed. Thus a small group of experienced endoscopists become experts in passing the tube, and this may account for the low complication rate in the Cape Town series [1]. The tube is inserted via the mouth and when well within the stomach, the gastric balloon is inflated with 200 ml of air. The tube is pulled back until the gastric balloon is sited firmly against the oesophagogastric junction. Traction is maintained and the tube held in place using a split tennis ball firmly strapped to the tube at the patient's mouth. This maintains effective tamponade at the oesophagogastric junction. Tension should be checked regularly at the mouth. Thereafter the oesophageal balloon is inflated to 40 mm Hg using a three-way tap and a Baumanometer. The gastric lumen is used for suction and to instil medication such as lactulose and neomycin. The fourth lumen (Boyce modification) is placed on constant suction to keep the oesophagus clear of secretions.

The patient is nursed in an intensive care unit and carefully monitored. A flat radiograph of the abdomen is taken at the bedside to check the position of the tube and will demonstrate the airfilled gastric balloon *in situ*.

A period of 6–24 hours is allowed for adequate resuscitation prior to taking the patient to the operating theatre for injection sclerotherapy. Furthermore, injection sclerotherapy can be planned as a definitive semielective procedure at a convenient time.

INJECTION SCLEROTHERAPY

The Cape Town experience [1]

In a five-year analysis, 66 patients had 137 separate variceal bleeds during 93 admissions to hospital in which initial Sengstaken tube tamponade was required for temporary control of variceal haemorrhage and which was followed by injection sclerotherapy. A total of 127 emergency injections were performed in this group of patients. There were 51 males and 15 females and the average age on first admission was 47 years (range: 13–80 years). The modified Child's risk grade [14] at the time of their initial admission was Grade A, 14; Grade B, 30; and Grade C, 19 (the grading was not estimated in three patients). Of the patients, 83% had cirrhosis (55% alcoholic cirrhosis, 24% cryptogenic cirrhosis and 4% cirrhosis plus carcinoma), 9% had portal vein thrombosis and the remaining 8% (five patients) consisted of two with congenital hepatic fibrosis, one with normal liver histology and two in whom the diagnosis was not established.

Variceal haemorrhage was controlled temporarily by the Sengstaken tube in all 137 bleeding episodes. Using the combination of Sengstaken tube and subsequent injection sclerotherapy, ultimate control of variceal haemorrhage was achieved in 95% of hospital admissions (88 of 93 admissions).

In 70% of hospital admissions, variceal haemorrhage was controlled with a single injection. In 22% of admissions, two or three injections were required, while one patient required four injections. No patient was subjected to more than four injections to achieve control.

The mortality per hospital admission in this group was 28% (26 deaths during 93 admissions). The mortality per variceal bleed was 19%. The causes of death are shown in Table 3.2. It is important to emphasize that no patient died of continued uncontrolled variceal bleeding.

Complications occurred on 22 occasions in 18 patients during the 93 admissions.

They are detailed elsewhere [1]. Despite these excellent results there is a small group of patients in whom variceal bleeding is difficult to control and where repeated bleeds lead to progressive liver failure and death. A recent reanalysis of the data has indicated that patients who require more than two injections to achieve control of haemorrhage during a single admission have a very high mortality. Other non-medical measures, such as portacaval shunts, are currently recommended in this small sub-group of patients (unpublished data).

Thus, in summary, definitive control of variceal haemorrhage was achieved in 95% of hospital admissions, usually with a single injection (70%). The mortality per hospital admission was 28%. No patient died of continued variceal bleeding and exanguinating variceal haemorrhage no longer poses a major problem in our hospital. The combined use of initial Sengstaken tube tamponade followed by injection sclerotherapy has simplified the emergency treatment in patients who present with continued active variceal bleeding, despite initial conservative treatment.

Table 3.2 Causes of death: 26 patients during 93 admissions [1]

Cause of death	Number of patients
Liver failure	21
Primary liver failure	5
Associated multiple organ failure	14
Associated Terminal variceal bleed	2
Complications of treatment	3
Sengstaken tube	2
Oesophagoscopy and injection	1
Cardiorespiratory	2
Uncontrolled variceal haemorrhage	0

Cape Town technique of rigid endoscopic sclerotherapy

Full technical details are presented elsewhere [1, 12]. After the Sengstaken tube has been passed and bleeding arrested temporarily, the patient is resuscitated and rendered as fit as possible for a general anaesthetic. Clotting defects are sought and corrected if possible. Patients are taken to the operating theatre at a convenient time ranging from 6–24 hours after insertion of the Sengstaken tube.

In the operating theatre, the Sengstaken tube is only removed after the patient has been anaesthetized and when the surgeon is ready to pass the oesophagoscope.

Patients are premedicated with atropine (0.6 mg) and diazepam (5–10 mg), unless the patient is stuperose or unconscious. Anaesthesia is induced with thiopentone sodium and suxamethonium, an endotracheal tube is inserted, and anaesthesia is maintained with nitrous oxide and oxygen, intermittent thiopentone plus intermittent suxamethonium or alloferrin. The procedure usually lasts 20–40 minutes.

The modified 50 cm long, wide bore, rigid Negus oesophagoscope with a slot at the distal end [15] is shown in Fig. 3.1. The scope is passed to the oesophagogastric junction as soon as the Sengstaken tube has been removed. Bleeding rarely recurs at this time, but if it does, it can be immediately controlled when the oesophagoscope reaches the oesophagogastric junction. With the modified Negus oesophagoscope, only one varix protrudes into the slot, while the other variceal channels are compressed. Each channel is injected with 6–8 ml of ethanolamine oleate, administered intravascularly into the varix, with the injection being sited just above the oesophagogastric junction. Sodium morrhuate is an alternative sclerosant which has been used in the USA [16, 17].

After injection of the first varix, immediate rotation of the oesophagoscope compresses that varix, trapping the sclerosant in position and preventing bleeding and loss of sclerosant from the needle prick site. At the same time a second varix presents in the slot, ready for injection. Usually three variceal channels require injection and are sited at two, six and ten o'clock (with the patient lying on his back).

At the end of the procedure, the oesophagoscope is left *in situ* for an arbitrary further five minutes to provide further compression and is then removed. The Sengstaken tube should not be replaced at the end of the procedure as it is unnecessary and can be either dangerous or difficult to insert.

The patient is returned to a surgical intensive care unit for 24–48 hours. Feeding is commenced with oral fluids during the first 24 hours followed by full feeding thereafter.

The advantages of using the rigid oesophagoscope have been published previously [11, 18]. This oesophagoscope has a proximal light source which does not become obscured if bleeding occurs. Only one distended varix projects into the slot of the oesophagoscope which is situated at the distal end opposite the beak. This facilitates injection. At the same time other variceal channels are compressed by the wide-bore oesophagoscope. After injection of the first varix, immediate rotation of the oesophagoscope compresses this varix, which promotes sclerosis and prevents bleeding or loss of sclerosant from the needle-prick site. At the same time the next varix presents for injection. Thereafter the third and any additional varices are similarly individually injected while compressing the already injected varices. In the authors' opinion the fibreoptic oesophagoscope, as presently designed, does not offer any of these advantages.

Fig. 3.1 The 50 cm rigid Negus oesophagoscope, the injection needle (below) and the suckers. Note that the needle and the suckers are offset at the proximal end. The slot at the distal end of the oesophagoscope is shown in the inset.

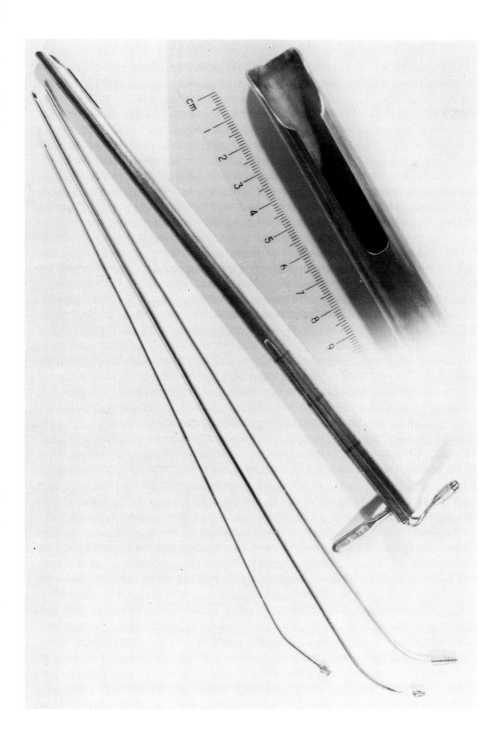

Other experience with rigid endoscopic sclerotherapy

Intravariceal injection was first reported by Crafoord and Frenckner in 1939 [19]. Initial interest was limited. The paper by Macbeth in 1955 [20] transiently rekindled interest, but it was the description of the excellent results of Johnston and Rodgers of Belfast [21] which marked the beginning of the modern era of endoscopic sclerotherapy. They controlled acute variceal haemorrhage in 93% of admissions (217 injections in 117 patients) over a 15-year period with a very low mortality (18% admission mortality). It should be noted that a quarter of their patients were in the better risk group with extrahepatic portal vein obstruction. A technique similar to that used by the Cape Town group has also been successfully used by Johnson [22], Bailey and Dawson [15], Barsoum *et al.* [23], Lilly [16] and Palani *et al.* [17].

ALTERNATIVE TECHNIQUES OF INJECTION SCLEROTHERAPY

Injection sclerotherapy may be performed directly, intravascularly into the varix, as detailed above, with the aim of thrombosing the varix and preventing further bleeding. An alternative technique, which is popular on the continent of Europe, is to inject the solution submucosally adjacent to the varix producing submucosal oedema which is reputed to prevent early rebleeding and subsequently to thicken the mucosa to prevent later rebleeding [24, 25].

Intravascular injection sclerotherapy has been performed using a fibreoptic scope by a number of authors. Unfortunately, some workers have used techniques which require a general anaesthetic. This removes a major advantage of using the fibreoptic scope. An example is the technique developed by the Kings College Hospital, London group which encorporates a flexible sheath over the fibreoptic scope [26, 27]. Other groups have modified the fibreoptic scope to incorporate balloons to achieve compression. These may either be attached to the oesophagoscope itself [28] or be sited distal to the oesophagoscope [29]. Both of these techniques can be performed without an anaesthetic and merit further evaluation. The most widely used technique today is to inject sclerosant directly into the varices via a fibreoptic endoscope without balloon compression [30]. Whether this method will be more successful than the rigid endoscope technique described above for managing acute variceal bleeding has still to be demonstrated and requires prospective controlled trials.

Submucosal injection sclerotherapy adjacent to the varix has been widely practised in Europe [24, 25]. Excellent results have been reported with the largest series being that of Paquet. In a recent report he had a 93% success rate in 305 patients with acute variceal bleeding [31].

For the past two years the Cape Town group have been comparing the rigid oesophagoscope technique using a general anaesthetic with a fibreoptic scope technique combining intravascular and submucosal injections without an anaesthetic in a prospective randomized controlled clinical trial.

OTHER FORMS OF TREATMENT

The case for Sengstaken tube tamponade and injection sclerotherapy in patients with continued acute variceal bleeding as opposed to other techniques has been presented in detail elsewhere [12, 32].

Percutaneous transhepatic obliteration of varices in the radiology department has been proposed as a valuable alternative form of therapy. A number of reports have appeared in the literature with the best results being achieved by Viamonte and colleagues [33]. They were successful in all 32 patients treated for acute variceal bleeding. Smith-Laing *et al.* were successful in 37 of 52 patients with active variceal bleeding [34], while Gembarowicz and colleagues were only successful in 50% of 20 patients who failed to respond to vasopressin [35]. Others have also noted failure of the technique [36, 37, 38]. Indeed, the group from Lund in Sweden who, originated the technique [39], and who have considerable experience with various modifications, have emphasized its problems and no longer advocate the procedure for acute variceal bleeding. The major problems have been portal vein thrombosis (36%), a high rebleed rate (55%) and difficulty in repeating the procedure in long term treatment [36]. Portal vein thrombosis, a very serious complication, has also been noted by other workers [37, 40].

The authors do not believe that emergency portosystemic shunting operations [41, 42] or devascularization and transsection procedures, which have been associated with a very high mortality in the past, are justified when a simple measure such as injection sclerotherapy is so successful. The major operations should probably be reserved for the rare failures of injection sclerotherapy. For the same reason, despite good results reported from Japan, the massive devascularization and transsection of Sugiura [43], also seems unjustified. Another new form of treatment has been oesophageal transsection using a stapling gun via the abdominal route [44, 45, 46]. Longer follow up and further published results are required to evaluate the true place of this procedure. However, problems in the setting of the treatment of acute variceal bleeding have been noted by one of the proponents [44, 47].

CONCLUSIONS

Patients with suspected oesophageal variceal bleeding require emergency endoscopy to prove, as far as possible, that varices are the source of their bleeding. Further measures should not be undertaken unless bleeding continues despite simple treatment, including intravenous pitressin infusion. Where bleeding continues, a correctly sited Sengstaken tube will stop the variceal bleeding temporarily. Major or dangerous procedures are unjustified when emergency peroesophageal injection sclerotherapy will ensure definitive control of variceal bleeding in 95% of cases. The more complex procedures should be reserved for the rare failures of injection sclerotherapy. Although the authors favour rigid endoscopy under general anaesthesia, a number of fibreoptic techniques, which can be used without general anaesthesia, are being evaluated. Controlled trials are required to determine whether they are as successful as the rigid endoscopic techniques.

ACKNOWLEDGEMENTS

This study was supported by grants from the South African Medical Research Council and the Staff Research fund of the University of Cape Town. Drs M. Jonker, H. Yakoob, R. Bane, D. Kahn, J. Northover and J. Wright have played a major role in the treatment and documentation of the patients and their assistance is acknowledged. The Medical Superintendent, Groote Schuur Hospital is thanked for permission to publish patient details.

REFERENCES

1. Terblanche, J., Yakoob, H. I., Bornman, P. C., Stiegmann, G. V. *et al.* (1981) Acute bleeding varices: a five-year prospective evaluation of tamponade and sclerotherapy. *Ann. Surg.*, **194** (4), 521–30.
2. Sagar, S., Harrison, I. D., Brearley, R. and Shields, R. (1979) Emergency treatment of variceal haemorrhage. *Br. J. Surg.*, **66**, 824–6.
3. Barr, J. W., Larkin, R. C. and Rosch, J. (1975) Similarity of arterial and intravenous vasopressin on portal and systemic hemodynamics. *Gastroenterology*, **69**, 13–19.
4. Chojkier, M., Groszmann, R. J., Atterbury, C. E., Bar-Meir, S. *et al.* (1979) A controlled comparison of continuous intraarterial and intravenous infusions of vasopressin in hemorrhage from esophageal varices. *Gastroenterology*, **77**, 540–6.
5. Johnson, W. C., Widrich, W. C., Ansell, J. E., Robbins, A. H. and Nabseth, D. C. (1977) Control of bleeding varices by vasopressin: A prospective randomised trial. *Ann. Surg.*, **186**, 369–76.
6. Novis, B. H., Duys, P., Barbezat, G. O., Clain, J. *et al.* (1976) Fibreoptic endoscopy and the use of the Sengstaken tube in acute gastrointestinal haemorrhage in patients with portal hypertension and varices. *Gut*, **17**, 258–62.
7. Chojkier, M. and Conn, H. O. (1980) Esophageal tamponade in the treatment of bleeding varices. A decadal progress report. *Dig. Dis. Sci.*, **25**, 267–72.
8. Conn, H. O. and Simpson, J. A. (1967) Excessive mortality associated with balloon tamponade of bleeding varices. *JAMA*, **202**, 587–91.
9. Agger, P., Anderson, J. R. and Burcharth, F. (1978) Does the oesophageal balloon compress oesophageal varices? *Scand. J. Gastroenterol.*, **13**, 225–7.
10. Johansen, T. S. and Baden, H. (1973) Re-appraisal of the Sengstaken-Blakemore balloon tamponade for bleeding esophageal varices: Results in 91 patients. *Scand. J. Gastroenterol.*, **8**, 181–3.
11. Terblanche, J., Northover, J. M. A., Bornman, P., Kahn, D. *et al.* (1979) A prospective evaluation of injection sclerotherapy in the treatment of acute bleeding from esophageal varices. *Surgery*, **85**, 239–45.
12. Terblanche, J. (1981) in *Advances in Surgery*, (ed. L. D. MacLean), Year Book Medical Publishers Inc., Chicago, pp. 257–91.
13. Boyce, H. W. Jr. (1962) Modification of the Sengstaken-Blakemore balloon tube. *New Engl. J. Med.*, **267**, 195–6.

14. Terblanche, J., Northover, J. M. A., Bornman, P. C., Kahn, D. *et al.* (1979) A prospective controlled trial of sclerotherapy in the longterm management of patients after esophageal variceal bleeding. *Surg. Gynecol. Obstet.*, **148**, 323–33.

15. Bailey, M. E. and Dawson, J. L. (1975) Modified oesophagoscope for injecting oesophageal varices. *Br. Med. J.*, **2**, 540–1.

16. Lilly, J. R. (1981) Endoscopic sclerosis of esophageal varices in children. *Surg. Gynecol. Obstet.*, **152**, 513–14.

17. Palani, C. K., Abuabara, S., Kraft, A. R. and Jonasson, O. (1981) Endoscopic sclerotherapy in acute variceal hemorrhage. *Am. J. Surg.*, **141**, 164–8.

18. Terblanche, J. (1979) Treatment of oesophageal varices (Editorial). *J. R. Soc. Med.*, **72**, 163–6.

19. Crafoord, C. and Frenckner, P. (1939) New surgical treatment of varicose veins of the oesophagus. *Acta Otolaryngol. Stockh.*, **27**, 422–9.

20. Macbeth, R. (1955) Treatment of oesophageal varices in portal hypertension by means of sclerosing injections. *Br. Med. J.*, **2**, 877–80.

21. Johnston, G. W. and Rodgers, H. W. (1973) A review of 15 years' experience in the use of sclerotherapy in the control of acute haemorrhage from oesophageal varices. *Br. J. Surg.*, **60**, 797–800.

22. Johnson, A. G. (1977) Injection sclerotherapy in the emergency and elective treatment of oesophageal varices. *Ann. R. Coll. Surg.*, **59**, 497–501.

23. Barsoum, M. S., Khattar, N. Y. and Risk-Allah, M. A. (1978) Technical aspects of injection sclerotherapy of acute oesophageal variceal haemorrhage as seen by radiography. *Br. J. Surg.*, **65**, 588–9.

24. Paquet, K.-J. and Oberhammer, E. (1978) Sclerotherapy of bleeding oesophageal varices by means of endoscopy. *Endoscopy*, **10**, 7–12.

25. Wodak, E. (1979) Akute gastrointestinale blutung; resultate der endoskopischen sklerosierung von osophagusvarizen. *Schweiz. Med. Wschr.*, **109**, 591–4.

26. Clark, A. W., Macdougall, B. R. D., Westaby, D., Mitchell, K. J. *et al.* (1980) Prospective controlled trial of injection sclerotherapy in patients with cirrhosis and recent variceal haemorrhage. *Lancet*, **ii**, 552–4.

27. Williams, K. G. D. and Dawson, J. L. (1979) Fibreoptic injection of oesophageal varices. *Br. Med. J.*, **2**, 766–7.

28. Brooks, W. S. (1980) Adapting flexible endoscopes for sclerosis of oesophageal varices. *Lancet*, **i**, 266.

29. Lewis, J., Chung, R. S. and Allison, J. (1980) Sclerotherapy of esophageal varices. *Arch. Surg.*, **115**, 476–80.

30. Harris, O. D., Dickey, J. D. and Stephenson, P. M. (1982) Simple endoscopic injection sclerotherapy of oesophageal varices. *Aust. NZ J. Med.*, **12**, 131–5.

31. Paquet, K.-J. (1981) in *Liver Update 1/81*, (eds R. E. Kirsch, M. Sherman and J. Terblanche), A.A. Balkema, Rotterdam, pp. 91–109.

32. Terblanche, J. (1981) in *More Controversies in Surgery*, (eds R. L. Varco and J. P. Delaney), W. B. Saunders and Co., Philadelphia, pp. 139–46.

33. Viamonte, M., Pereiras, R., Russell, E., Le Page, J. and Hutson, D. (1977) Transhepatic obliteration of gastroesophageal varices. Results in acute and nonacute bleeders. *Am. J. R.*, **129**, 237–41.

34. Smith-Laing, G., Scott, J., Long, R. G., Dick, R. and Sherlock, S. (1981) Role of percutaneous transhepatic obliteration of varices in the management of hemorrhage from gastroesophageal varices. *Gastroenterology*, **80**, 1031–6.

35. Gembarowicz, R. M., Kelly, J. J., O'Donnell, T. F., Millan, V. A. *et al.* (1980) Management of variceal hemorrhage. Results of a standardized protocol using vasopressin and transhepatic embolization. *Arch. Surg.*, **115**, 1160–4.

36. Bengmark, S., Borjesson, B., Hoevels, J., Joelsson, B. *et al.* (1979) Obliteration of esophageal varices by PTP. A follow-up of 43 patients. *Ann. Surg.*, **190**, 549–54.

37. Henderson, J. M., Buist, T. A. S. and MacPherson, A. I. S. (1979) Percutaneous transhepatic occlusion for bleeding oesophageal varices. *Br. J. Surg.*, **66**, 569–71.
38. Scott, J., Long, R. G., Dick, R. and Sherlock, S. (1976) Percutaneous transhepatic obliteration of gastro-oesophageal varices. *Lancet*, **ii**, 53–5.
39. Lunderquist, A. and Vang, J. (1974) Transhepatic catheterization and obliteration of the coronary vein in patients with portal hypertension and esophageal varices. *New Engl. J. Med.*, **291**, 646–9.
40. Passariello, R., Thau, A., Lombardi, M., Simonetti, G. and Stipa, S. (1980) Control of gastroesophageal bleeding varices by percutaneous transhepatic portography. *Surg. Gynecol. Obstet.*, **150**, 155–60.
41. Malt, R. A., Abbot, W. M., Warshaw, A. L., Vander Selm, T. J. and Smead, W. L. (1978) Randomized trial of emergency mesocaval and portacaval shunts for bleeding esophageal varices. *Am. J. Surg.*, **135**, 584–8.
42. Orloff, M. J., Bell, R. H., Hyde, P. V. and Skivolocki, W. P. (1980) Long-term results of emergency portacaval shunt for bleeding esophageal varices in unselected patients with alcoholic cirrhosis. *Ann. Surg.*, **192**, 325–40.
43. Sugiura, M. and Futagawa, S. (1977) Further evaluation of the Sugiura procedure in the treatment of esophageal varices. *Arch. Surg.*, **112**, 1317–21.
44. Johnston, G. W. (1982) Six years' experience of oesophageal transection for oesophageal varices, using a circular stapling gun. *Gut*, **23**, 770–3.
    stapling gun. *Gut*, **23**, 770–3.
45. Takasaki, T., Kobayshi, S., Muto, H., Suzuki, S. *et al.* (1977) Transabdominal esophageal transection by using a suture device in cases of esophageal varices. *Intern. Surg.*, **62**, 426–8.
46. Wexler, M. J. (1980) Treatment of bleeding esophageal varices by transabdominal esophageal transection with the EEA stapling instrument. *Surgery*, **88**, 406–16.
47. Johnston, G. W. (1981) Bleeding oesophageal varices: The management of shunt rejects. *Ann. R. Coll. Surg.*, **63**, 3–8.

4

Laser photocoagulation

PAUL SWAIN

THE NATURE OF THE PROBLEM

In the UK, 30 000 patients are admitted every year with acute upper gas-trointestinal haemorrhage and nearly 3000 (nearly 10%), will die as a consequence of the bleeding [1]. There is little evidence that the mortality rate has changed over the last 25 years despite the more accurate diagnostic information provided by endoscopy and improvements in intensive medical and surgical therapy [2, 3, 4]. Rebleeding following hospital admission is the most important bad prognostic factor [5] and if this could be reduced by non-operative means, the high mortality from the complications of emergency surgery might be avoided. The finding of a 'visible vessel' in an ulcer crater also carries a high risk of rebleeding and offers a specific target for endoscopic therapy [6, 7].

A potential non-operative means of preventing rebleeding is laser photocoagulation. The main advantages of laser therapy over rival endoscopic techniques such as diathermy are that the bleeding point is not touched or disturbed mechanically during therapy and the amount of energy dissipated in the surrounding tissue is more easily predicted and controlled.

THE LASER AND ITS HISTORY

The word 'laser' (light amplification by the stimulated emission of radiation) is among the most successful of acronyms to enter the English language. There are three types of laser commonly in use in medicine: Argon in ophthalmology and dermatology; Nd YAG in experimental surgery and carbon dioxide used in surgery as a knife (gynaecology, laryngology and neurosurgery). At present only argon and Nd YAG beams can be passed down flexible waveguides suitable for endoscopic use in clinical gastroenterology.

The principles of stimulated emission was predicted by Einstein as early as 1917. During the 1950s Townes in Columbia University and Basov and Prokhorov in the Lebedev Institute who were working independently in the field of microwave physics, applied the theory of quantum mechanics to demonstrate that stimulated emission of radiation could be made available for practical use. They received the Nobel Prize for this work in 1964. The first practical laser was reported in Nature by Maiman working for the Howard Hughes Aircraft Corporation in 1960 and was a pulsed ruby laser [8]. Both types of laser currently used in gastroenterology were invented in the early 1960s [9, 10].

As early as 1974 two German groups described the passage of the argon laser via an endoscopic wave guide. The argon laser emits radiation energy in the visible blue green range of the spectrum (wavelength $0.44-0.52\,\mu$m). The beam is focused onto the tip of a thin flexible quartz fibre and exists from the distal tip of the wave guide with a small degree of divergence (about $10°$). A small amount of laser light is used to aim the laser beam onto the bleeding point before it is fired at full power.

Several groups have reported the results of studies to evaluate the safety and effectiveness of argon laser photocoagulation in controlling bleeding of experimental gastric ulcers in animals [13, 14]. Their conclusions are summarized here. Effective haemostasis using the argon laser has definitely been demonstrated for animal model gastric ulcers. Power should be greater than 5 watts for 90% successful haemostasis while the depth of damage (perforation risk) is much greater at 12 watts than at 9 watts without significant improvement in haemostasis. The argon laser's effectiveness is limited in severe bleeding because it can be absorbed by red blood gushing from a bleeding lesion rather than by the underlying vessel that is the real target for coagulation. The use of a stream of inert gas, [15] usually carbon dioxide, coaxial to the laser beam may remove the overlying blood allowing the laser energy to be deposited on the bleeding vessel and also helps to clear secretions from the tip and cool it. This restricts the maximum treatment distance, best results being obtained 5–15 mm from the lesion. Endoscopic gastric overdistension has to be avoided which is not only uncomfortable for the patient but increases the depth of tissue damage for a given amount of laser power. The gas is usually vented via the biopsy channel in a two-channel endoscope, or via a nasogastric tube passed alongside a conventional one-channel endoscope, though an ingenious fail safe gas recycling system has been recommended [16]. The carbon dioxide markedly lessens the small risk or intracolonic gas explosion if the laser is used in conjunction with colonoscopy. High power treatment of a small spot, i.e. high energy density, which means power per unit/per unit area will produce an erosive effect drilling a hole which can perforate vessels and cause haemorrhage rather than coagulation.

INTERACTION OF LASER LIGHT WITH BIOLOGICAL TISSUE

The most important interaction of laser radiation with tissue is the absorption of the light by the tissue with the consequent conversion of the light energy to heat at the point or small area where the laser beam hits the tissue.

The effect of heat on tissue varies with the temperature achieved. Between 37°C and 60°C simple heating occurs with a consequent speeding of temperature-dependent enzyme reactions and altered water permeability characteristics, between 60–70°C denaturation of protein occurs with loss of cell membrane integrity and alterations in the form of structural proteins. At 100°C boiling of tissue water occurs causing cells to explode, and at higher temperatures carbonization with charring is observed. The observed effects are those seen in heating a piece of steak with slight local swelling as membrane integrity is lost, the appearance of opalescence as proteins lose their tertiary structure, contraction mainly due to alterations of fibrous tissue proteins, the crackling or spitting as cells swell and explode, dehydration and further loss of volume as evaporation takes place and charring with loss of mechanical strength as the temperature exceeds 100°C followed by vaporization to steam and carbon particles and finally catching fire.

It remains uncertain which of these effects is responsible for the coagulation properties of heat. Vessel shrinkage is probably important in producing initial instantaneous haemostasis. It has been doubtfully suggested that local oedema disturbing the patency of the bleeding vessel may be of importance. Heat damage to vascular endothelium may activate the coagulation cascade and produce secondary intravascular thrombosis, but histology suggests that this may take hours to develop while the usual effect on experimental bleeding ulcers is instantaneous.

There is a limit to the size of external vessel that can be occluded by either laser. Vessels greater than 1.5 mm in diameter are sealed with increasing difficulty, although small holes in large vessels such as the aorta can be reliably sealed without occluding the whole vessel. The matrix in which the vessel lies and in particular the amount of contractable fibrous tissue in proximity to the vessel probably also contribute to the effectiveness of haemostasis.

The ultimate tissue effect produced depends on both temperature developed in the tissue and duration of laser exposure. But the different radiation tissue absorption characteristics of Nd YAG and argon laser energy are responsible for important differences in histological effect [13]. Nd YAG radiation tissue absorption is low compared to argon while scattering of the light energy in all directions is much more significant. This scattering of Nd YAG radiation leads to an affected area much greater in diameter than the beam, especially as the depth increases. Argon laser radiation has a high absorption coefficient so the intensity of the light energy drops off rapidly as the beam passes deeper into the tissue and is particularly absorbed by red pigment which means that a thin film of blood, or a spurt from a vessel may absorb the energy, preventing it from reaching and sealing the hole in the vessel that is responsible for bleeding.

CLINICAL EXPERIENCE WITH ARGON LASER PHOTOCOAGULATION

Several groups have reported using the argon laser in patients since the first description of the endoscopic use in man by Frühmorgen in 1974 from Erlangen [17]. He has more recently described approximately 300 lesions in 100 patients, reporting success rates of 95%, although this included some rebleeds who were subsequently coagulated [18]. The technique appears to be relatively safe and perforations have not yet been reported by groups using this technique. Two other uncontrolled studies reported successful stopping of bleeding rates at 86% (Brunetaud) [19] and 80% (Cotton) [20]. It must be remembered that these apparently successful uncontrolled studies in patients have been carried out in a condition where the spontaneous cessation of bleeding rate is of the order of 85–90%, and although these series have variously selected out 'high risk' patients, the efficacy of this treatment required testing by controlled clinical trials and two randomized trials have been reported this year.

Vallon [21] reported the results of a trial carried out in Barcelona. Of 332 patients admitted with upper gastrointestinal bleeding, 136 had peptic ulcers. Of these, 28 were bleeding actively at endoscopy. The actively bleeding ulcers were randomized to sham or argon laser therapy. Of 15 laser treated bleeding ulcers, ten stopped bleeding (67%). Of 13 control patients four stopped (31%). The results approach the 5% level of statistical significance. Of the 15 deaths in patients admitted to the trial, five were in laser treated patients and ten in controls, suggesting a trend favouring the argon laser although this difference was not statistically significant due to the small number of patients entered. These workers felt that there was little evidence that the argon laser prevented rebleeding in a patient with a non-bleeding peptic ulcer with a red spot or 'visible vessel' in its crater, although their numbers show a small non-significant trend favouring the laser.

We [22] have recently reported the results of a controlled trial carried out in two London hospitals. Of 330 consecutive admissions for upper gastrointestinal bleeding, 155 patients were found to have ulceration as a cause. Of these all 76 patients having 'stigmata of recent haemorrhage' i.e. a visible vessel, red spots or adherent clot in the base of an ulcer, were included in the trial if accessible to laser therapy. Stratification was in three groups: ulcers with a visible vessel (52 total, 11 actively spurting); those without a vessel, but with red or black spots (17); those with an overlying clot persisting after washing (seven). Of the 52 patients with a visible vessel, eight out of 20 treated and 17 out of 28 controls had further haemorrhage ($P < 0.05$). No treated patients but 7 control patients died ($P < 0.02$).

We concluded that argon laser photocoagulation reduced the incidence of rebleeding and the mortality rate in patients admitted with acute gastrointestinal bleeding when endoscopy has revealed an ulcer with a visible vessel in its base.

NEODYMIUM YTTRIUM ALUMINIUM GARNET (Nd YAG) LASER

At effective haemostasis energy levels the depth of penetration of this invisible laser beam with a wavelength of 1.06μm in the near infra-red spectrum is greater than the argon. Although the Nd YAG laser is absorbed by haemoglobin, this absorption is far less efficient than with argon and its energy is more widely scattered, is mostly absorbed by water and tissue proteins and is converted to heat. This may make haemostasis more effective in the presence of rapid haemorrhage (a relatively uncommon endoscopic problem) than with the argon laser, but it increases the depth of injury and risk of perforation. Studies in experimental canine gastric ulcer have established that optimum power levels are between 50–90 watts and with exposure times of 0.3–0.7 seconds for haemostasis without full thickness damage [23, 24]. There is however an obvious discrepancy between the acute experimental canine gastric ulcer and the chronic gastric or duodenal ulcer where not only the mucosa is lost, but also the submucosa and usually the muscularis mucosa and a hard mat of fibrous connective tissue is often stuck to adjacent organs. The difference in optimum power levels (for argon 8 watts for 1–3 s and for Nd YAG 80 watts for 0.3–0.5 s) may be explained as follows: the Nd YAG laser heats approximately three times larger volume of tissue than does an equal energy density derived from an argon laser and so requires a greater amount of energy to raise the temperature comparably to achieve photocoagulation.

CLINICAL EXPERIENCE WITH THE Nd YAG LASER

Kiefhaber and Nath in Munich have had very extensive practical experience in treating patients with gastrointestinal bleeding with Nd YAG [25]. They have treated more than 600 patients and have reported results on 110 patients claiming to stop bleeding in 93% of cases, and include treatment of 40 patients with bleeding oesophageal varices. A German firm that makes Nd YAG lasers report that in Germany more than 1000 patients have been treated with this therapy in a number of German centres since 1975 and report an observed perforation incidence of 1%. In Kiefhaber's series two perforations occurred in cases that were treated with the laser on the same spot on consecutive days in acute (i.e. thin-walled) ulcers. There is a need for studies on post-mortem and surgically resected specimens to assess depth of damage in man.

The largest controlled trial of Nd YAG laser photocoagulation has been reported this year from Vantrappen and Rugeerts [26] in Brussels in abstract form. Of 227 patients in their trial they were able to stop 100% of bleeding lesions and have shown a significant reduction in rebleeding rate but not yet in mortality rate. Results from smaller studies and controlled trials, some of which are still in progress including Ihre [27], Rohde, Escorrou [28], McLeod and our own have not yet produced definitive results, but probably none have yet put through the very large numbers of suitable patients required to demonstrate clear cut effects on mortality and bleeding rates.

In summary the results of the first laser photocoagulation trials are most encouraging but not yet definitive. It is to be hoped that with more experience the results may improve further. The total impact of lasers on the problem of gastrointestinal bleeding remains to be assessed, but it has to be accepted that not all bleeding lesions treated are immune from further haemorrhage particularly if a large vessel is exposed in an ulcer. There are several clinical questions yet to be answered. What are the best power levels and exposure times for use in the chronic human ulcer? They could be higher since the ulcer's base will reflect more light energy backwards. Is it better to attempt to obliterate the lumen of the bleeding vessel or simply seal a hole in it with a single perfectly aimed shot? Is it worth repeating laser therapy if a patient bleeds again? Are lasers more effective, more cost effective or safer than electrocoagulation?

PRACTICAL PROBLEMS

Laser safety [27]

The main theoretical risk to the patients is that of perforating a viscus. This has not yet been reported with argon and the reported incidence with Nd YAG users seems acceptably low and may improve now that safe parameters have been delineated. Other complications include occasionally starting bleeding (fortunately this usually settles spontaneously unless spurting is observed). Discomfort from gaseous overdistension and sometimes protracted endoscopy may occur. Metal laser tips are occasionally dropped inside patients' stomachs, but will emerge in the stool without sequelae. The main risk to the operator or to others in the room during endoscopy is of inadvertent eye damage – one endoscopist has already reported causing a scotoma on his retina using the Nd YAG laser [28]. Although both lasers are 'class four lasers', in other words potentially capable of causing eye damage before the eye has time to blink, the Nd YAG laser may be more dangerous than the argon since its light energy is in the invisible part of the spectrum, and therefore the eye will not tend to blink when it is fixed and also because it scatters more (up to 40%) of the light energy in a backwards direction, i.e. back towards the endoscopist's eye. Many safety systems are currently used, either marketed by the firms making the lasers or devised by hospital laser safety officers; none are foolproof but effective protection can be relatively easily maintained with responsible usage, and current experience suggests that laser usage is not likely to produce a generation of one-eyed endoscopists.

The problems that will be involved in installing a laser in a gastrointestinal unit will include finance. Laser systems currently cost between £30 000–60 000. They will require a three-phase electrical supply, some requiring high voltage. A high-flow water cooling system may have to be plumbed in, and this may occasionally flood the endoscopy room floor. Because of the electric and water supply, lasers are not portable at present and patients have to be moved to the laser.

To maintain acceptable power outputs some laser systems require periodic maintenance, particularly to tune up the optical performance. The main technical problems of using lasers with endoscopes relate to the fragility of current generation of wave guides. The commonest cause of tip destruction is forgetting to turn the coaxial gas on, or the cylinder running out during use and unexpected contact of the gut wall with the laser tip when it is fixed. This is usually associated with a characteristic smell of burnt plastic coming up from the patient. Replacement fibres for some systems are expensive, costing from £200–500, some have the advantage that you can cut off the end and fit a new tip yourself.

Both argon and Nd YAG lasers are being used with carbon dioxide gas jet systems and the gas needs to be removed in some way to prevent over-distension. We sometimes use a two-channel endoscope with one channel to pass the laser wave guide and the second to remove the gas but sometimes pass a small-bore nasogastric tube down by the side of a conventional smaller one-channel endoscope which may allow for greater manoeuvrability. Not all laser systems can pass through the small 2.2 mm biopsy channel in 'paediatric' endoscopes, although now 2.8 mm channel paediatric diameter endoscopes are available. Some laser systems require that an endoscope be dedicated to laser use, to have an optical safety filter inserted into the eyepiece and a wave guide cut to its particular length.

Recent studies have suggested that laser photocoagulation is effective in controlling recurrent haemorrhage from both hereditary haemorrhagic telangiectasiae and angiodysplasia, diminishing the need for transfusion, surgery and hospital admission [31, 32]. Lasers have been used down endoscopes to destroy gastrointestinal tumours, some Japanese groups have used them to destroy early gastric cancers [33] and they have been found effective in the palliative relief of symptomatic obstruction in the oesophagus [34] and stomach [35] in cases where surgical relief could not be undertaken. Gallstones in the common duct have recently been destroyed endoscopically in a few patients [36, 37].

In the rapidly expanding field of therapeutic endoscopy laser photocoagulation seems to offer new grounds for optimism that gastrointestinal bleeding may be controlled by non-surgical means, and that the mortality rate may be reduced.

REFERENCES

1. Allan, R. and Dykes, P. (1976) A study of the factors influencing mortality rates from gastrointestinal haemorrhage. Q. J. Med., New Series XLV, 533–50.

2. Schiller, K. F. R., Truelove, S. C. and Williams, G. D. (1970) Haematemesis and melaena with special reference to factors influencing the outcome. *Br. Med. J.*, **2**, 7–14.

3. Peterson, W. L., Barnett, C. C., Smith, H. J., Allen, M. H. and Corbett, D. B. (1981) Routine early endoscopy in upper gastrointestinal tract bleeding: a randomised controlled trial. *New. Engl. J. Med.*, **304**, 925–9.

4. Conn, H. O. (1981) To scope or not to scope. *New Engl. J. Med.*, **304**, 967–9.

5. Avery-Jones, F. (1956) Haematemesis and melaena with special reference to causation and to the factors influencing the mortality from bleeding peptic ulcers. *Gastroenterology*, **30**, 166–9.

6. Griffiths, W. J., Neumann, D. A. and Welsh, J. D. (1979) The visible vessel as an indicator of uncontrolled or recurrent gastrointestinal haemorrhage. *New Engl. J. Med.*, **300**, 411–13.

7. Storey, D. W., Brown, S. G., Swain, C. P., Salmon, P. R. *et al.* (1981) Endoscopic prediction of recurrent bleeding in peptic ulcers. *New Engl. J. Med.*, **305**, (16), 915–16.

8. Maiman, T. H. (1960) Stimulated optical radiation in ruby. *Nature*, **187**, 493–4.

9. Kahida, E. F., Gordon, F. I. and Miller, R. C. (1965) Continuous duty argon ion lasers. *IEEE J. Quantum Electron.*, **1**, 273–9.

10. Gensic, J. E., Marcos, H. M. and van Uitert, L. G. (1964) Laser oscillations in Nd-doped yttrium aluminium, yttrium gallium and gadolinium garnet. *Appl. Phys. Lett.*, **4**, 182–4.

11. Nath, G., Gorish, W. and Kiefhaber, P. (1973) First laserendoscopy via a fibreoptic transmission system. *Endoscopy*, **5**, 208–13.

12. Frühmorgen, P., Reidenbach, H. R., Bodem, F. *et al.* (1974) Experimental examinations on laser endoscopy. *Endoscopy*, **6**, 116–22.

13. Silverstein, F. E., Protell, R. L., Piercy, J., Rulin, C. E. *et al.* (1977) Comparison of the efficacy of high and low power photocoagulation in control of severely bleeding experimental ulcers in dogs. *Gastroenterology*, **73**, 481–6.

14. Bown, S. G., Salmon, P. R., Kelly, D. F., Calder, B. M. *et al.* (1979) Argon laser photocoagulation in the dog stomach. *Gut*, **20**, 680–7.

15. Silverstein, F. E., Protell, R. C., Gulacsik, C., Auth, D. C. *et al.* (1978) Endoscopic laser treatment III. The development and testing of a gas-jet-assisted argon laser wave guide in control of bleeding experimental ulcers. *Gastroenterology*, **74**, 232–9.

16. Auth, D. C., Gulacksik, C., Silverstein, F. E., Rubin, C. R. *et al.* (1978) A clinically useful endoscopic laser coagulator with recirculating gas jet assistance. Presented at the Conference on Laser and Electro-Optical Systems, San Diego.

17. Frühmorgen, P., Bodem, F., Reidenback, H. D. *et al.* (1976) Endoscopic laser photocoagulation of bleeding gastrointestinal lesions with report of the first therapeutic application in man. *Gastrointest. Endosc.*, **23**, 73–5.

18. Frühmorgen, P., Bodem, F., Reidenbach, H. R., Kaduk, B. and Demling, L. (1978) Endoscopic photocoagulation by laser irradiation in the gastrointestinal tract of man. *Acta Hepatogastroenterol. (Stuttgart)*, **25**, 1–5.

19. Brunetaud, J. M., Enger, A., Flamert, J. B. *et al.* (1979) Utilisation d'un laser a argon conisé en endoscopie digestive: photocoagulation des lesion hemorragiques. *Rev. Phys. Appl.*, **19**, 385.

20. Laurence, B. H., Cotton, P. B., Vallon, A. G. *et al.* (1980) Endoscopic laser photocoagulation for bleeding peptic ulcers. *Lancet*, **i**, 124–5.

21. Vallon, A. G., Cotton, P. B., Laurence, B. H., Armengol Miro, J. R. *et al.* (1981) Randomised trial of endoscopic argon laser photocoagulation in bleeding peptic ulcers. *Gut*, **22**, 228–33.

22. Swain, C. P., Bown, S. G., Storey, D. W., Northfield, T. C. (1981) Controlled trial of argon laser photocoagulation in bleeding peptic ulcers. *Lancet*, **ii**, 1313–16.

23. Bown, S. G., Salmon, P. R., Storey, D. W., Calder, B. A. *et al.* (1980) Nd-YAG laser photocoagulation in the dog stomach. *Gut*, **21**, 818–25.

24. Dixon, J. A., Berenson, M. M. and McClosky, D. W. (1979) Neodymium-YAG laser treatment of experimental canine gastric bleeding. *Gastroenterology*, **77**, 647–51.
25. Kiefhaber, P., Nath, G. and Moritz, K. (1977) Endoscopic control of massive gastrointestinal haemorrhage by irradiation with a high power Nd-YAG laser. *Prof. Surg.*, **15**, 140–55.
26. Vantrappen, G., Rutgeerts, P., Broeckaert, L., Jenssens, J. and Coremans, C. (1981) Controlled trial of Nd-YAG laser treatment for upper digestive haemorrhage. *Gastrointest. Endosc.*, **27**, 139.
27. Ihre, T., Johansson, C., Seligsen, U. and Torrigren, S. (1981) Endoscopic YAG laser treatment in massive upper gastrointestinal bleeding. Report of a controlled randomised study. *Scand. J. Gastroenterol.*, **16**, 633–40.
28. Escourrou, J., Frexinos, J., Bommelaer, G., Edouard, R. *et al.* (1981) Prospective randomised study of YAG photocoagulation in gastrointestinal bleeding: *Laser Tokyo*, **5**, 30.
29. Mallow, A. and Chabot, L. (1978) *Laser Safety Handbook*, Van Ristrand Reinhold Company, New York.
30. Becker, C. D. (1977) An accident victims view. *Laser Focus*, **August**.
31. Jensen, D. M., Machicado, G. A., Tapia, J. I., Beclin, D. B. and Mautner, W. (1981) Endoscopic treatment of haemangiomata with argon laser in patients with gastrointestinal bleeding. *Laser Tokyo*, 20–5.
32. Jensen, D. M., Machicado, G. A., Tapia, J. I., Beclin, D. B. and Mautner, W. (1981) Argon laser photocoagulation of bleeding colonic lesions. *Laser Tokyo*, 20–4.
33. Imaoka, W., Okuda, J., Ida, K. and Kawai, K. (1981) Treatment of digestive tract tumour with laser endoscopy – experimental and clinical studies. *Laser Tokyo*, 5–7.
34. Fleishcer, D. (1981) Palliative therapy for esophageal carcinoma by endoscopic Nd-YAG laser. *Laser Tokyo*, 20–17.
35. Swain, C. P., Bown, S. G., Edwards, D. W. and Salmon, P. R. (1981) Neoplastic gastric outflow tract obstruction relieved by argon laser at endoscopy. *Laser Tokyo*, 5–32.
36. Hayakawa, N., Nimura, Y., Kamiya, J., Hasegawa, H. *et al.* (1981) Studies on laser cholangioscopy – application for lithotripsy of gall stones. *Laser Tokyo*, 23–16.
37. Orii, K., Takase, Y., Ozaki, A., Okamura, T. *et al.* (1981) Lithotomy of bile duct stone by YAG laser with a choledochofiberscope. *Laser Tokyo*, 23–16.

5

Endoscopy in portal hypertension

P. M. SMITH and J. D. R. ROSE

WHY DO VARICES BLEED?

Variceal haemorrhage is related to variceal size and not to portal pressure, once portal hypertension is well established [1]. Large tortuous varices are, therefore, more likely to bleed than small ones. Haemorrhage seems to be explosive in nature through a pin-hole in the vein, and not erosive. Mucosal lesions overlying bleeding sites are seldom seen [2], and excess gastro-oesophageal reflux does not occur in patients with variceal bleeding [3]. Re-bleeding rates do not seem to be affected by Child's grading [4], but continued heavy alcohol intake predisposes to further haemorrhage.

WHERE DO VARICES BLEED FROM?

Bleeding occurs from an oesophageal varix within 2 cm of the gastro-oesophageal junction. Blood loss above or below this level is uncommon. Although the King's College Hospital Group [5] attributed bleeding to a gastric varix in 21% of their cases, this has not been the experience of other workers. We found only two out of 49 patients to have bled from gastric varices; the remaining 47 lost blood from the lower end of the oesophagus.

TECHNIQUE OF FIBREOPTIC SCLEROTHERAPY

After spraying the throat with lignocaine, intravenous Diazemuls (emulsified diazepam), sufficient to produce dysarthria or ptosis, precedes passage of an end-viewing fibrescope with the patient in the left lateral position. Buscopan (hyoscine butyl bromide) is used to paralyse the oesophagus. The new wide-bore biopsy channel instruments provide better suction facilities should haemorrhage occur, but an endoscope with a bridge (Olympus GIFD 4) allows more accurate placement of the injection needle. No outer sheath [6] is used. Using a fine injection needle (Olympus NM 3), 2 ml of sodium tetradcyl sulphate is injected into each varix just above the gastro-oesophageal junction and the patient is returned to the ward. If variceal bleeding is precipitated, which is rare in our experience, then a Sengstaken tube is passed for four hours. Further injections are performed weekly until variceal size has decreased, and with it the risk of bleeding, and thereafter are continued at monthly intervals on a day admission basis until all varices have been obliterated. We have found that between two and 13 treatments are required, depending on the initial variceal size.

Since the direction of blood flow in the varix is upwards, treatment confined to the lower 5 cm of the gullet is sufficient to eradicate oesophageal bleeding. Persistence of varices further up the gullet in a few patients has not given rise to any problems and they may be safely ignored.

CLASSIFICATION OF VARICES

Variceal size is assessed subjectively and graded I to IV, according to our own criteria, which, however, correspond to those recently published by Paquet [7]. After passage of a thin plastic tube down the biopsy channel, a few drops of water are injected to facilitate orientation. The direction of fall of the drops is taken to be six o'clock, and the position of varices is noted on a clock face system at 30, 35 and 40 cm, so that the progress of individual varices can be followed (Fig. 5.1). A variceal score can be derived from the sums of the variceal grades immediately above and 5 cm proximal to the gastro-oesophageal junction. Photographs are taken for reference purposes.

WHICH SCLEROSANT?

In Britain sodium tetradcyl sulphate (STD) and ethanoleamine oleate (EO) are used, whereas on the Continent hydroxy-poly-ethoxy dodecanoic acid (HPD) is favoured. The work of Blenkinsopp [8, 9] on the effect of sclerosants on rat femoral veins demonstrated that STD was superior to EO and equal in potency to HPD. STD and EO produced similar degrees of tissue necrosis when injected subcutaneously, but HPD was less likely to produce ulceration. EO is more viscous than STD, which is particularly important when trying to inject it down a long fine needle. EO is also irritant if sclerosant sprays into the eyes. We therefore prefer STD.

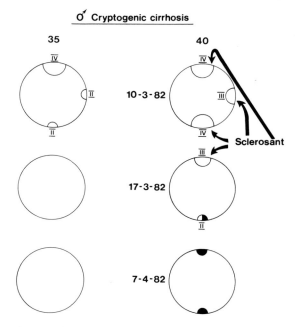

Fig. 5.1 Progress of sclerotherapy. Varices recorded and graded to demonstrate thrombosis and reduction in size.

Most sclerosants are detergents, and animal work suggests that contact with the vein endothelium for one second only is sufficient to produce irreversible maceration [10] and thrombosis [11]. Furthermore, the sclerosants retain their surfactant properties even when considerably diluted [12]. Transient exposure of the endothelium of the varix to sclerosant is, therefore, effective.

IS COMPRESSION OF THE VARIX HELPFUL?

The role of compression devices, such as the Williams' tube [6], remains controversial. They have the theoretical advantages of trapping the sclerosant within the vein for longer, of lessening bleeding after sclerotherapy and, by distending the vein, making it easier to inject. On the other hand, a general anaesthetic may be required; the tube itself has caused perforation; and it makes orientation within the oesophagus more difficult. Furthermore, since brief contact of the sclerosant with the vein endothelium is sufficient to produce thrombosis [11], compression is unnecessary. Westaby and his colleagues [13] found an increased elimination of varices with the Williams' sheath, but the difference just failed to reach statistical significance, the trial was not double blind, and the advantage was valid only for the second sclerotherapy session.

Balloons have also been used to achieve compression above [14] or below [15, 16] the site of injection, but the published results do not appear to be superior to those achieved by simple fibreoptic sclerotherapy [17].

RE-BLEEDING DURING TREATMENT

The danger of re-bleeding before variceal obliteration is achieved is greatest early in treatment while the varices are still large (grade III or IV; Fig. 5.2). Patients with multiple large varices require more injections to achieve sclerosis than those with small varices (grades I and II), the number of injections correlating with the variceal score (Fig. 5.3) and are therefore at risk of re-bleeding for a longer period of time. No patient of ours with small varices only has bled during treatment, except for one with a sclerosant-induced ulcer. In comparison, 10 out of 13 patients who had three or more large varices re-bled. This suggests that a patient with multiple large varices should be treated as often as possible to achieve obliteration before re-bleeding occurs. We do not advise that sclerotherapy should be performed more than once every four days; although thrombosis occurs within hours, the ulceration that can follow extravasation of the sclerosant may take a

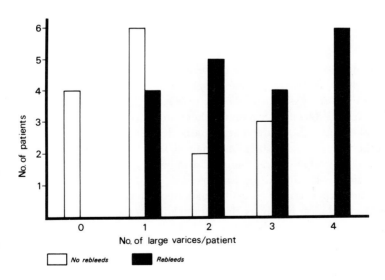

Fig. 5.2 Relationship of numbers of large varices present initially to rebleeding. Difference in number of large varices between re-bleeding and non-rebleeding groups is significant. $p = <0.01$, Mann-Whitney U test. (With permission from *Gut* [26].)

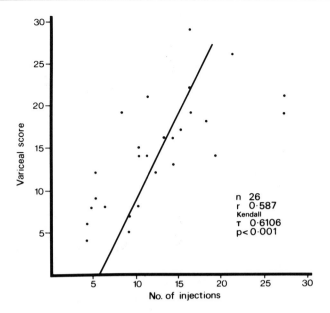

Fig. 5.3 Correlation between initial variceal score and number of injections required to obliterate varices. (With permission from *Gut* [26].)

week to develop [18]. It is often convenient to inject weekly until the varices have become small, and thereafter monthly until they are gone. Disappearance depends on fibrosis of the vascular channels, which may take several weeks [19].

The acutely bleeding varix is difficult to inject, and we prefer to rely on a Sengstaken tube for initial haemostasis. If recurrent bleeding renders further sclerotherapy impracticable, oesophageal transection with a stapling gun [20] provides a period of several months during which follow-up sclerotherapy can be used to deal with any variceal recurrence. We have not found that transection alone leads to permanent cure. One patient of ours was found at operation to have a longitudinal ulcer involving the full thickness of the oesophageal wall, following an injection of sclerosant four days earlier; the necrotic tissue was excised and the varices successfully ligated.

We believe that the cirrhotic with bad liver function should not be allowed to have more than one major bleed. Hepatic decompensation with coma and ascites may follow haemorrhage. In addition, coagulation difficulties can follow large blood transfusions. Oesophageal transection should be considered after a blood loss of four pints or more, or whenever a Sengstaken tube fails to arrest bleeding.

WHERE SHOULD THE SCLEROSANT BE INJECTED?

Although most British endoscopists aim to inject the sclerosant intravenously, paravasal treatment of vascular anomalies has existed since the 1970s. Wodak [21] developed the concept of ösophaguswandsklerosierung – oesophageal wall sclerosis – whose aim was to bury the varices in a thick protective fibrous coat by multiple submucosal injections of sclerosant. A modification of this technique is paravasal injection, in which the sclerosant is injected next to the varix. Although one group [22] have reported no benefit from a technique they described as paravasal, no direct comparison of injections into or next to varices has been made. To do this, a contrast-sclerosant mixture of 3% STD and 76% urografin in a 1:3 ratio was injected and radiological control was used to identify the site of injection (Figs 5.4 and 5.5). Two groups of 10 varices were injected, one intravariceally, the other paravariceally. Intravariceal contrast vanished rapidly but paravasal contrast was visible for up to 90 minutes. Despite this prolonged action it was ineffective, for when the varices were examined one month later only three out of the paravasal group were thrombosed compared with eight of the intravariceal group (Fig. 5.6). One paravasal injection produced an ulcer which bled.

Using the same radiological technique further studies were performed to assess how frequently an intended intravariceal injection was in fact paravariceal. Of 59 intended intravariceal injections, whose site could be accurately identified radiologically, 15 were paravasal (25%). Large varices were successfully entered in 82% (31/38) of injections compared with 62% (13/21) for small varices.

Since it is impossible for the endoscopist to aspirate blood up the injection needle with the syringe at the time of treatment, he cannot check that the needle is in the vein without X-ray screening, so the chance of extravascular injection of sclerosant increases as the vein becomes smaller. A proportion of injections are, therefore, less effective because the sclerosant is not intravenous, although paravasal injection may thrombose some small varices.

Ten patients had their varices obliterated under radiological control, using 0.5 ml of the sclerosant contrast mixture to demonstrate the site of injection and only giving a full injection when the needle was intravariceal. The results in these ten were compared to those obtained for 29 patients treated earlier by the conventional free hand technique (Figs 5.7 and 5.8). There was a more rapid reduction in variceal size, a significant reduction in the number of injection sessions required, and no strictures developed. This suggests that free hand injection is less effective because it is not always intravariceal, and extravasated sclerosant is not of benefit.

Paquet [23] has produced oesophageal wall sclerosis by multiple (30–40) submucosal injections of dilute sclerosant, repeated on 2–4 occasions, to produce a protective fibrous sheath around the varices. His results are impressive and the complication rate is acceptably low, although 1.7% developed necrosis of the oesophageal wall with mediastinitis or empyema [24]. The use of a small volume of

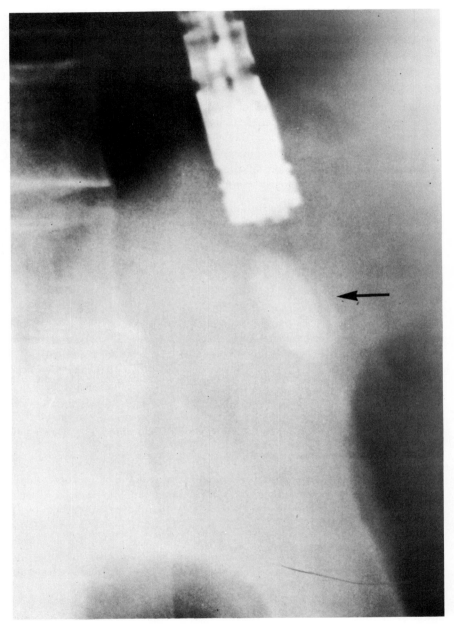

Fig. 5.4 Radiological demonstration of paravasal injection.

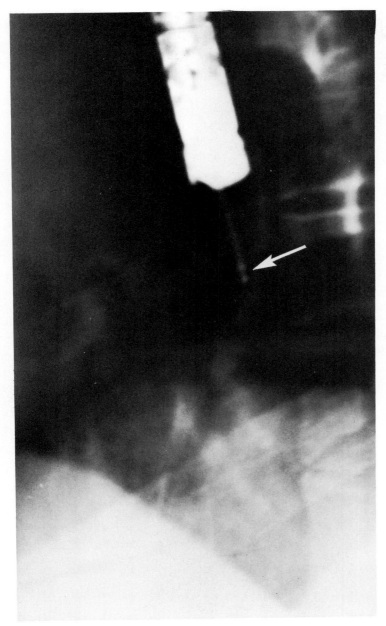

Fig. 5.5 Radiological demonstration of intravariceal injection.

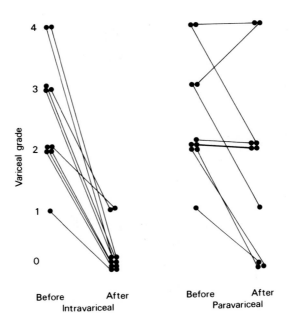

Fig. 5.6 Results of intravariceal and paravariceal injection. Grade 0 is no varix visible or varix thrombosed. Thrombosis in intravariceal group is significantly higher. $p = 0.032$, Exact test. (With permission from *Gut* [26].)

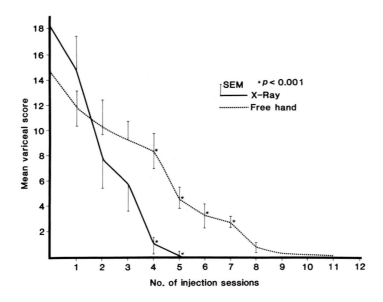

Fig. 5.7 Effect of radiological control on variceal score reduction.

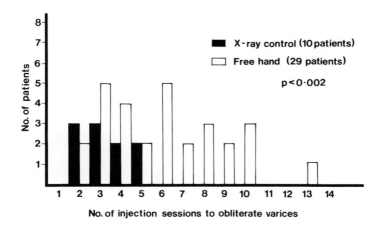

Fig. 5.8 Effect of radiological control on number of sessions required to obliterate varices.

dilute sclerosant is undoubtedly responsible for the low incidence of complications. However, other workers have not been able to produce such good results [22].

GASTRIC VARICES

It has been argued that thrombosis of the oesophageal varices will lead to an increase in portal hypertension and bleeding from gastric varices. However, we have shown by injecting sclerosant contrast mixture into oesophageal varices under radiological control, that gastric varices fill from above (Fig. 5.9).

Varices at the cardia have, therefore, not been a problem since it has been possible to sclerose them from the oesophagus. The fact that they fill so readily from above may mean that these varices are extensions of oesophageal varices rather than their supplying vessels, which lie deeper in the gastric wall.

COMPLICATIONS OF FIBREOPTIC SCLEROTHERAPY

Bleeding is rarely precipitated by sclerotherapy, unless coughing or struggling (usually in an alcoholic) lead to a variceal laceration by the injection needle. In the uncomplicated patient, no more than a few drops of blood are lost on withdrawal of the needle. Instrumental perforation should not occur, although occasional cases have followed the use of the Williams' over tube or a rigid endoscope [25].

Other complications are related to the extravascular injection of sclerosant, confirmed by our radiological studies of the site of injection of sclerosant contrast

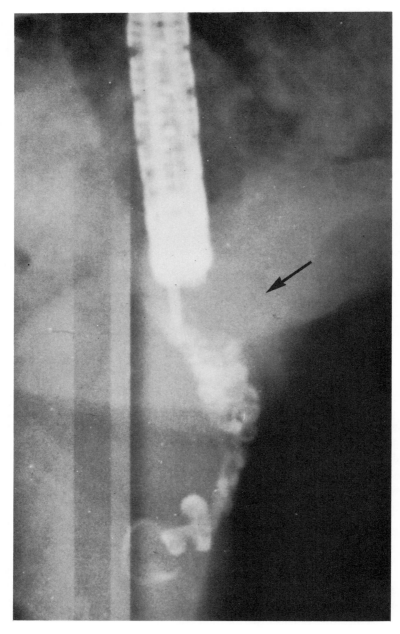

Fig. 5.9 Radiological demonstration of filling of a gastric varix from an oesophageal injection.

mixture. Intravenous injection gave rise to no complications in a series of 10 patients; of 10 paravasal injections, one produced dysphagia and another an ulcer that bled [26]. Substernal pain is common for 48 hours after treatment. It resolves quickly and responds to alkalies. Oesophageal ulcers have been reported in 11–27% of patients [15, 25, 26]. They heal within a month and may be symptomless. The radiological pattern of paravasal injection suggests that they result from sclerosant spreading along the vein sheath, ulcerating the overlying mucosa. Occasionally, the ulceration may even penetrate the vein walls to produce haemorrhage.

Whereas a single misplaced injection of sclerosant may result in an oesophageal ulcer, multiple injections (3–7) are required to produce an oesophageal stricture and submucosal fibrosis (Fig. 5.10). Using free hand injection techniques, strictures have been seen in 16–27% of successfully treated patients [17, 25], the development of the stricture coinciding with the disappearance of the varices. In some patients the stricture will spontaneously resolve, in others one or two dilatations by the Eder–Puestow technique [27] will suffice.

More serious complications can occur. Pyrexia may follow oesophageal tissue necrosis, and oesophageal perforation, empyema, pleural effusions, oesophageal aortic fistulae and broncho-oesophageal fistulae [28] have also been described.

Careful techniques, including radiological screening and the use of small volumes of sclerosant should avoid many of these problems, however. The development of a less toxic but equally effective sclerosant would be helpful.

DOES FIBREOPTIC SCLEROTHERAPY WORK?

The various controlled trials of portacaval shunting have shown that the decreased risk of bleeding is matched by an increased mortality and morbidity from porta-systemic encephalopathy and liver failure [29, 30]. In contrast, sclerotherapy does not affect liver blood flow or function. It is, therefore, not surprising that controlled trials of sclerotherapy have shown improved survival [25, 31, 32]. The largest trial so far reported is from King's College Hospital [25]. Only four patients out of 42 bled after variceal obliteration during a mean follow-up period of 14 months, whereas 42 out of 56 patients in the control group bled during a mean follow-up of 9.5 months; a highly significant difference. The overall risk of bleeding per patient month of follow-up was reduced threefold by sclerotherapy. Unfortunately, the underlying liver disease is not affected by sclerotherapy, so patients continue to die. During our follow-up of 39 successfully treated patients over a period of 1–40 months (mean 21), 8 have died, 3 from hepatic failure, 1 each from hepatoma, bronchopneumonia and septicaemia, and 2 from gastric bleeding.

DO VARICES RECUR?

Of our 39 patients 10 developed recurrent varices during a mean follow-up period of 21 months after successful sclerotherapy. Of these 10, only two bled, in neither

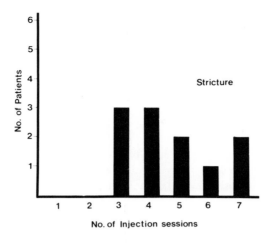

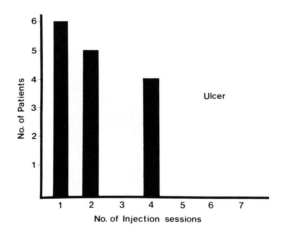

Fig. 5.10 Time of first appearance of complications.

case seriously, one and two months after the last endoscopy. The recurrences were seen during the first year, but there have been none in the 15 patients followed for more than 12 months (Fig. 5.11). A second recurrence also took place in half the relapsed patients, one as late as 20 months after a second obliteration. Similar figures were obtained by the King's College Hospital Group [25] with 15 variceal recurrences in 42 successfully treated patients during a mean follow-up period of 9 months. In 13 of these the recurrence was detected at routine follow-up endoscopy,

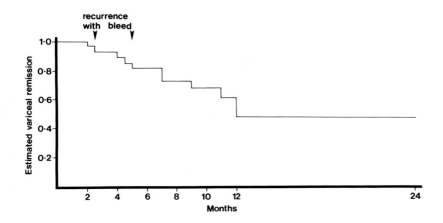

Fig. 5.11 Life-table analysis of variceal remission in 39 patients.

and only 2 patients presented with further bleeding 8 and 13 months after initial obliteration. Paquet, who uses the paravasal sclerotherapy technique, had to re-inject 40% of his patients every year to treat recurrent varices [24].

We have re-endoscoped our patients at three monthly intervals after variceal obliteration for the first year, extending follow-up to six monthly for the second and third year. If all is well, then thereafter check endoscopies need be performed only annually.

Current knowledge suggests that follow-up should be indefinite, but some patients seem to go into prolonged remission. In our series there are four patients with a mean variceal remission of 26 months. Although it would be premature to talk of a cure Paquet [33] considers a 'Dauererfolg' – continued success – possible in 50% of his patients.

PROPHYLACTIC SCLEROTHERAPY

What should be done with oesophageal varices that have not bled? Paquet [7] has treated patients whom he considered to be of high risk because they have grade III–IV varices with overlying erosions, or grade II–IV varices with coagulation factors below 30%. In the treated group the mortality was 6% over a two year period, in comparison to a death rate of 42% for the control group. In Britain, however, with a lower incidence of alcoholic cirrhosis than in Germany, the mortality of a similar control group would be much lower and the indications for prophylaxis are not clear cut. It is our policy to treat only grade III and grade IV varices if we think there is a real chance of bleeding within the next few months. Further controlled trials are required to confirm Paquet's results.

CONCLUSION

Fibreoptic sclerotherapy will obliterate varices and prolong survival. The technique is simple and can be performed without compression devices or general anaesthesia. Large varices require more injections than small varices for obliteration, and re-bleeding during treatment occurs only in patients with large varices.

Radiological studies have shown that intravariceal sclerosant is significantly more effective than paravasal injections. Extravasated sclerosant is probably responsible for the complications of the technique, of which ulceration and stricture formation are commonest. The use of radiological screening techniques reduces the incidence of complications and the number of injections required for obliteration.

Follow-up to detect recurrent varices should be three monthly in the first year after obliteration, but can be six monthly thereafter.

ACKNOWLEDGEMENTS

Dr M. D. Crane helped with the radiological studies, and Mr M. H. Wheeler performed the oesophageal transections.

REFERENCES

1. Lebrec, D., De Fleury, P., Rueff, B., Nahum, H. and Benhamou, J. P. (1980) Portal hypertension, size of esophageal varices and risk of gastrointestinal bleeding in alcoholic cirrhosis. *Gastroenterology*, **179**, 1139–44.
2. Orloff, M. J. and Thomas, H. S. (1963) Pathogenesis of esophagus varix rupture. A study based on gross and microscopic examination of the esophagus at the time of bleeding. *Arch. Surg.*, **87**, 301–7.
3. Eckhardt, V. F. and Grace, N. D. (1979) Gastroesophageal reflux and bleeding esophageal varices. *Gastroenterology*, **76**, 39–42.
4. Westaby, D., MacDougall, B. R. D., Saunders, J. B. and Williams, R. (1982) in *Variceal Bleeding* (eds D. Westaby, B. R. D. MacDougall and R. Williams), Pitman Books, London, pp. 21–33.
5. Mitchell, K., Theodossi, A. and Williams, R. (1982) in *Variceal Bleeding* (eds D. Westaby, B. R. D. MacDougall and R. Williams), Pitman Books, London, pp. 62–5.

6. Williams, K. G. D. and Dawson, J. L. (1979) Fibreoptic injection of oesophageal varices. *Br. Med. J.*, **2**, 766–7.
7. Paquet, K-J. (1982) Prophylactic sclerosing treatment of the esophageal wall in varices – a prospective controlled randomized trial. *Endoscopy*, **14**, 4–5.
8. Blenkinsopp, W. K. (1968) Comparison of tetradecyl sulphate of sodium with other sclerosants in rats. *Br. J. Exp. Pathol.*, **49**, 197–201.
9. Blenkinsopp, W. K. (1970) Choice of sclerosant: An experimental study. *Angiologica*, **7**, 182–6.
10. Dietrich, H. P. and Sinapius, D. (1968) Experimentelle Endothelschädigung durch Varizenverödungsmittel. *Anzneimittelforschung*, **18**, 116–20.
11. Blenkinsopp, W. K. (1968) Effect of injected sclerosant (Tetradecyl Sulphate of Sodium) on rat veins. *Angiologica*, **5**, 386–96.
12. Rose, J. D. R. Unpublished observations.
13. Westaby, D., MacDougall, B. R. D., Theodossi, A., Melia, W. and Williams, R. (1982) Prospective randomized study of two techniques of injection sclerotherapy. *Gut*, **23**, 450.
14. Scott Brooks, W. (1980) Adapting flexible endoscopes for sclerosis of oesophageal varices. *Lancet*, **i**, 266.
15. Lewis, J., Chung, R. S. and Allison, J. (1980) Sclerotherapy of esophageal varices. *Arch. Surg.*, **115**, 476–80.
16. Kirkham, J. S. and Quayle, J. B. (1982) Oesophageal varices; evaluation of injection sclerotherapy without general anaesthesia using the flexible fibreoptic gastroscope. *Ann. R. Coll. Surg. Eng.*, **64**, 401–5.
17. Smith, P. M., Jones, D. B. and Rose, J. D. R. (1982) Simplified fibre endoscopic sclerotherapy for oesophageal varices. *J. R. Coll. Phys. Lond.*, **16**, 235–6.
18. Evans, D. M. D., Jones, D. B., Cleary, B. K. and Smith, P. M. (1982) Oesophageal varices treated by sclerotherapy: a histopathological study. *Gut*, **23**, 615–20.
19. Schneider, W. and Fischer, H. (1974) Histologie des varices sclérosées. *Phlebologie*, **27**, 411–6.
20. Johnston, G. W. (1982) Six years of experience of oesophageal transection for oesophageal varices, using a circular stapling gun. *Gut*, **23**, 770–3.
21. Wodak, E. (1960) Ösophagusvarizen – Blutung bei portaler Hypertension; ihre Therapie und Prophylaxe. *Wien. Med. Woch.*, **110**, 581–3.
22. EVASP Study Group (1982) Randomized trial of endoscopic sclerotherapy as a supplement to balloon tamponade for oesophageal varices. *Scand. J. Gastroenterol.*, **17** (Suppl. 78), 20.
23. Raschke, E. and Paquet, K-J. (1973) Management of hemorrhage from esophageal varices using esophagoscopic sclerosing method. *Ann. Surg.*, **177**, 99–102.
24. Paquet, K-J. (1982) in *Variceal Bleeding* (eds D. Westaby, B. R. D. MacDougall and R. Williams), Pitman Books, London, pp. 148–56.
25. MacDougall, B. R. D., Westaby, D., Theodossi, A., Dawson, J. L. and Williams, R. (1982) Increased long-term survival in variceal haemorrhage using injection sclerotherapy. *Lancet*, **i**, 124–7.
26. Rose, J. D. R., Crane, M. D. and Smith, P. M. (1983) Factors affecting successful endoscopic sclerotherapy for oesophageal varices. *Gut*, **24**, 946–9.
27. Price, J. D., Stanciu, C. and Bennett, J. R. (1974) A safer method of dilating oesophageal strictures. *Lancet*, **i**, 1141–2.
28. Carr-Locke, D. L. and Sidky, K. (1982) Broncho-oesophageal fistula; a late complication of endoscopic variceal sclerotherapy. *Gut*, **23**, 1005–7.
29. Conn, H. O. (1974) Therapeutic portacaval anastomosis: to shunt or not to shunt. *Gastroenterology*, **67**, 1065–71.

30. Rueff, B., Prandi, D., Degos, F., Sicot, J., Degos, J. D., Sicot, C., Maillard, J. N., Fauvert, R. and Benhamou, J. P. (1976) A controlled study of therapeutic portacaval shunt in alcoholic cirrhosis. *Lancet*, **i**, 655–9.
31. Terblanche, J., Northover, J. M. A., Bornman, P., Kahn, D., Silber, W., Barbezat, G. O., Sellars, S., Campbell, J. A. H. and Saunders, S. J. (1979) A prospective controlled trial of sclerotherapy in the long term management of patients with oesophageal variceal bleeding. *Surg. Gynecol. Obstet.*, **148**, 323–33.
32. Söderlund, C. (1982) Endoscopic sclerotherapy of bleeding oesophageal varices: a prospective controlled trial. *Scand. J. Gastroenterol.*, **17**, (Suppl. 78), 20.
33. Müting, D. (1982) in *Leber und Gallenwegserkrankungen* (D. Müting and R. Fischer), Schattauer Verlag, Stuttgart, p. 222.

6

Therapeutic radiology

D. J. ALLISON

Interventional radiology is useful in the management of both acute and chronic bleeding. In addition to standard diagnostic and therapeutic procedures, specialized techniques may be necessary in difficult cases, particularly in the search for microvascular abnormalities, and in the investigation and management of portal hypertension [1].

ACUTE BLEEDING

Angiography is used as a diagnostic measure in acute bleeding to localize the source of bleeding when previous endoscopy has failed to do this and the patient continues to bleed. In this situation angiography can detect blood loss in excess of 0.5 ml min^{-1}, and may be invaluable in guiding the surgeon to the site of pathology. Selective coeliac, superior mesenteric, and inferior mesenteric arteriograms will usually reveal the site of the bleeding but super-selective studies (e.g. gastroduodenal, left gastric, etc.) may be necessary in some circumstances. Once the site of bleeding (or a likely responsible lesion) has been demonstrated, the patient can then proceed to surgery if the bleeding continues. When the bleeding is from an anatomical site which is readily identifiable (e.g. stomach, caecum, etc.) no further radiological intervention is necessary unless surgery is contraindicated or inappropriate. If, however, the bleeding is from a site which may be difficult for the surgeon to locate at laparotomy (e.g. small bowel), then a catheter can be selectively inserted into the segmental artery supplying the actual lesion under fluoroscopic control in the angiographic unit. The patient is then transferred to the operating theatre with this catheter *in situ* and intraoperative angiography performed to localize precisely the abnormal area for the surgeon.

Angiography may also be used therapeutically in order to control bleeding without having recourse to surgery. This is achieved by:

(a) Drug (e.g. vasopressin) infusion through a selective catheter [2]. This technique is particularly useful in the case of diffuse bleeding such as haemorrhagic gastritis where surgery may be undesirable and embolization ineffective. Vasopressin infusion has also been used with great success in the control of bleeding of diverticula in the colon.

(b) Balloon catheters to obstruct flow to the bleeding site.

(c) Embolization. Emboli such as Sterispon, dura mater, or steel coils can be inserted into the bleeding vessel to arrest haemorrhage [3]. The technique of embolization has been used extensively in the management of gastrointestinal bleeding and is particularly useful in patients in whom operative surgery or general anaesthesia would be difficult or dangerous. Major branches in the coeliac territory such as the left gastric, hepatic, gastroduodenal, or gastroepiploic can be selectively embolized with very little risk of infarction of normal viscera owing to the rich collateral blood supply in the upper gastrointestinal tract. Ischaemic necrosis can occur however [4], and the risk of this is greatly increased if multiple simultaneous embolizations are performed, if there is pre-existing arterial disease, or if previous surgery has comprised the available collateral circulation. The method can be used to control acute bleeding from Mallory–Weiss tears, peptic ulcers, tumours, trauma, aneurysm, vascular malformations and iatrogenic bleeding due to recent biopsy or surgery [1, 5, 6]. It is more hazardous to embolize lesions in the lower gastrointestinal tract than in the stomach and duodenum because less reliance can be placed on the existence of adequate alternative arterial pathways, particularly in the splenic flexure and descending colon. Although there are case reports of successful colonic embolization, the procedure is probably inadvisable in most cases.

CHRONIC BLEEDING

In patients with chronic gastrointestinal bleeding in whom repeated investigations (e.g. endoscopy, barium studies, etc.) have failed to demonstrate any abnormality, angiography may demonstrate a vascular abnormality that is responsible for the bleeding. Some of these abnormalities may be exceedingly small and peroperative angiography is occasionally necessary to localize them, particularly in the small bowel. A common microvascular cause of bleeding in the large bowel is angiodysplasia [7, 8], and specialized postoperative studies of the resected bowel are required to localize the lesions for the pathologist. Embolization can also be used in the management of lesions causing chronic bleeding such as arteriovenous malformations and angiomas. It is probably not a suitable method for the treatment of angiodysplasia.

PORTAL HYPERTENSION

Vascular approaches may be used:

(a) To control or prevent bleeding from oesophageal varices by vasopressin (arterial or venous), or by direct embolization using the percutaneous trans-hepatic portal venous approach. Although embolization of varices with coils, isobutyl–2–cyanocrylate, ethanol and other agents is undoubtedly successful in the acute control of variceal bleeding, in most cases the benefit it confers may only be temporary. This is either because of the recanalization of embolized vessels or because of the appearance of new varices. The role therefore of therapeutic embolization in the management of patients with varices is controversial, particularly since endoscopic injection is now proving to be very successful. Details of the techniques of transhepatic variceal occlusion together with a review of the literature and an assessment of its current role can be found in the excellent article by Dick [9].

(b) To show the anatomy, patency and flow dynamics of the portal circulation prior to portocaval shunt. This may require indirect or direct (trans-splenic) portography.

(c) To demonstrate the patency of the hepatic veins by hepatic venography. This route may also be used to obtain hepatic vein wedge pressure and to perform transjugular hepatic biopsy [10].

CONCLUSIONS

Angiography plays an important role in the management of gastrointestinal bleeding because of its ability to detect extremely small vascular abnormalities and because of its important therapeutic applications. With the advent of digital vascular imaging systems, the development of safer and painless contrast media, and the increasing success of embolization methods, angiography seems likely to remain a significant diagnostic and therapeutic method in the management of bowel bleeding.

REFERENCES

1. Allison, D. J. (1980) Gastrointestinal bleeding. *Br. J. Hosp. Med.*, **358**, 23–4.
2. Athanasoulis, C. A. (1976) Arteriographic methods for the control of gastric haemorrhage. *Am. J. Dig. Dis.*, **21**, 174–81.
3. Allison, D. J. (1978) Therapeutic embolization. *Br. J. Hosp. Med.*, **20**, 707–16.
4. Goldman, M. L., Land, W. C., Bradley, E. L. and Anderson, J. (1976) Transcatheter therapeutic embolization in the management of massive upper gastrointestinal tract bleeding. *Radiology*, **120**, 513–21.

5. Reuter, S. R., Chuang, V. P. and Bree, R. L. (1975) Selective arterial embolization of control of massive upper gastrointestinal bleeding. *Am. J. Roentgenol.*, **125**, 119–26.
6. Katzen, B. T., Rossi, P., Passariello, R. and Simonetti, G. (1976) Transcatheter therapeutic arterial embolization. *Radiology*, **120**, 523–31.
7. Baum, S., Athanasoulis, G. A., Waltman, A. C., Galdabini, J. *et al.* (1977) Angiodysplasia of the right colon: a cause of gastrointestinal bleeding. *Am. J. Roentgenol.*, **129**, 789–94.
8. Boley, S. J., Sammartano, R., Adama, A., Dibiase, A. *et al.* (1977) On the nature and etiology of vascular ectasias of the colon. *Gastroenterology*, **72**, 650–60.
9. Dick, R. (1981) Transhepatic injection of varices. *Br. J. Hosp. Med.*, **26**, 340–7.
10. Allison, D. J. (1981) Therapeutic aspects of radiology. *Hosp. Update*, **7**, 851–71.

7

Recent advances in surgery

T. IHRE

THE DIFFICULT BLEEDING PATIENT

Severe upper gastrointestinal bleeding is present when the circulation is or has been affected. Any patient with severe upper gastrointestinal bleeding is a challenge to the treating physician or surgeon.

The initial caretaking of the patient has to be directed towards the following main lines:

(a) Re-establish circulation
(b) Diagnosis
(c) Careful supervision
(d) Treatment

'A difficult bleeding patient' can then be defined as one where one or many of these goals is not achieved.

RE-ESTABLISH CIRCULATION

In the majority of patients the bleeding will have stopped before the admission to the emergency ward and in these patients re-establishment is of no major difficulty. In a small number of patients the bleeding on admission is continuous and so severe that although massive transfusion is given the circulation is not properly restored. These bleedings are mostly caused by large arterial erosions as in duodenoaortal fistulas or massive bleeding from oesophageal varices. Our primary goal in these patients is to diagnose the bleeding source. The diagnostic procedure – endoscopy – should be performed under general anaesthesia with intubation to avoid aspiration and to enable maximal supervision of the patient. As severe bleedings and haematemesis in itself are a terrifying experience these patients are often difficult to deal with and the general anaesthesia might well be necessary when the endoscopy has to be performed.

During endoscopy a large tube is placed in the oesophagus, using the instrument as a guide. Through this tube suction can be performed which enables clearing the stomach from blood. If a visible bloodstream is seen to come from the duodenum we would, once oesophageal varices have been excluded, perform a laparotomy under the same anaesthesia. I will discuss later as to how to diagnose the bleeding source at an operation.

Oesophageal varices, which in our hospital in Stockholm is responsible for 25% of all severe upper gastrointestinal bleedings, are also best diagnosed with the tube in position. This tube will, in most cases, compress the varices once it has been pushed down a few centimetres below the cardia. Once the variceal bleeding has stopped the stomach and duodenum can be cleaned from blood and carefully inspected by endoscopy to exclude other bleeding sources. The tip of the endoscope is then placed at the oesophagogastric junction and the tube is pulled upwards. A side-viewing or oblique-viewing instrument will provide the best inspection of the varices. It is of course important to rotate the instrument tip 360°. A bleeding varix might be found but it is often difficult to find the exact bleeding spot even with this procedure and the diagnosis and treatment of the patients bleeding condition will then be based on other liver stigmata, the presence of varices and on exclusion of other bleeding sources.

DIAGNOSIS

Before the era of routine emergency endoscopies unnecessary laparotomies were performed in patients with oesophageal varices because of uncertainty of the bleeding source. Today the bleeding source with endoscopy is missed in some 3–5% of cases. Most of these patients will have stopped bleeding before endoscopy, but a small group of patients will have large amounts of fresh blood in their stomach. If oesophageal or gastric varices have been ruled out there are two other major causes of these bleedings that have to be born in mind: exulceratio simplex Dieulafoy and low duodenal ulcers. Exulceratio simplex Dieulafoy is a condition where the patient, without any previous history of ulcer disease, is bleeding from a large hypertrophic artery protruding from the mucosa without any ulcer present. The most common location is in the fundus which makes it even more difficult to diagnose. Many of these patients will bleed intermittently, but once they bleed their circulation rapidly becomes instable.

The condition is best diagnosed by endoscopy but angiography might also be useful. Excision or oversewing of the vessel is mostly sufficient as treatment. Recurrence has never been described once treatment has been given, but multiple lesions might be present.

Low duodenal ulcers, that is when the crater is situated in the region of, or below, the papilla of Vater are in our own experience often missed at endoscopy. These ulcers often involve the gastroduodenal artery and they therefore bleed massively and will need an emergency operation.

CAREFUL SUPERVISION

Supervising a patient who has a bleeding that has effected the circulation and who is anxious, is best done in the intensive care unit. If supervision is not done with all the facilities connected to the intensive care unit *then* you might easily have a difficult bleeding patient.

TREATMENT

The difficult bleeding patient in regard to treatment will be a patient where treatment is difficult because of unknown origin of the bleeding, or where the condition itself is incurable as in some cases of gastric cancer. Another kind of difficulty arises when the patient after initial successful treatment has a recurrent bleeding. I will concern myself with the very first item: the unknown origin of the bleeding source.

In patients with massive upper gastrointestinal bleeding where endoscopy has failed to reveal the source of bleeding the same indications for operation are present as in cases with a proven cause. If a laparotomy is performed we would start with a large gastrotomy along the greater curve of the stomach going down to the pyloric region. We would then, after cleaning the stomach from blood, put a tamponade down through the pylorus and one up the oesophagus and then carefully inspect the stomach. We often use a plastic tube with a diameter of 8 cm and the length of 20 cm through which inspection, suction and wiping can be done. This facilitates the inspection, especially of the fundus region. If no visible source of bleeding has been found in the stomach we would remove the tamponade in the pylorus and palpate down into the duodenum. Inspection of the duodenal cap and the descending duodenum is best done through either a sigmoidoscope or a proctoscope.

Then again, if there is no source of bleeding but blood is seen to come from below the duodenal cap, I would enlarge my gastrotomy and open the duodenum so that a direct inspection can be done. If finally still no bleeding source has been found, I would concentrate on the oesophagus even though I know that oesophagoscopy has been negative. I might inspect the oesophagus with an endoscope during the laparotomy, or have some one else do it.

This is how we would deal with these kind of patients. In 90–95% of cases we would find the cause of bleeding and then be able to treat it. Sadly there remains a very small group of patients where no bleeding source is found and who stop bleeding during operation, only to continue a few hours after the operation has been finished. Angiography can sometimes be of help but reoperation might also be necessary. We have, during the last three years, had one case in whom the bleeding source was never found, not even at the post mortem that followed after he had exsanguinated.

IN CONCLUSION

The difficult bleeding patient is so termed due mostly to the lack of diagnosis. The treatment is seldom of any difficulty, the exception being lack of effect of treatment, but that is another story altogether.

In order to decrease the number of the difficult patients we must get better at diagnosing and I suppose that is why we are all here.

8

The place of surgery in bleeding peptic ulcer

M. J. S. LANGMAN

Two basic beliefs underlie the management of acute bleeding from gastric or duodenal ulcers. These are:

(a) Early investigation by endoscopy will aid management.

(b) Individuals with ulcer bleeding, particularly if elderly, should be operated upon if bleeding recurs in hospital.

Evidence in support of these beliefs is indifferent, and experience in Nottingham suggests that both may be.ill-founded.

EARLY ENDOSCOPIC INVESTIGATION OF HAEMATEMESIS AND MELAENA

We have previously reported the initial results of a controlled trial in which patients with haematemesis or melaena were randomly allocated to groups investigated by radiology or endoscopy [1]. We have now expanded the data so that groups are sufficiently large to decide whether investigation does or does not affect the clinical outcome in acute upper gastrointestinal bleeding.

Method

Patients with acute upper gastrointestinal bleeding admitted to the two Nottingham University Hospitals which serve a population of some 700 000 people were randomly allocated at admission to investigation by barium meal radiography, using a double contrast technique, or to endoscopy. Investigation was usually conducted on the morning following admission and wherever possible patients who were investigated by one method were not reinvestigated by the other.

In all 1037 patients were entered in the trial; 336 were excluded, 110 because investigation was considered unnecessary, usually because bleeding was trivial in the context of the patient's general condition; 100 were unallocated due to failures of the randomization system, in 52 of these randomization could not be attempted at the weekends for part of the study time at one of the hospitals; 60 patients were considered unsuitable for radiography, 29 because of previous gastric surgery, 27 because a recent barium meal had been normal, and four because they were pregnant; in 26 further patients endoscopy was thought to be inappropriate because patients had severe cardiorespiratory disease, and five individuals refused investigation. Finally, in 27 patients early surgery was necessary before investigation was attempted and eight patients died soon after admission.

Results

The 526 patients randomly allocated to investigation by endoscopy and the 511 investigated radiologically proved generally comparable in terms of age and severity of bleeding.

The diagnostic yield was substantially higher in patients endoscoped than in those investigated radiologically, but the pattern of findings differed. This was partly because more superficial lesions were found endoscopically but also because more gastric ulcers were found endoscopically and more duodenal ulcers radiologically (Table 8.1).

The effect of investigation on patient management was assessed by examining operation rates, length of hospital stay, and mortality rates (Table 8.2). No differences of any note were detected, though patients endoscoped if they did come to operation tended to do so earlier than those examined radiologically. In those patients who died or came to operation the accuracy of diagnostic findings could be examined. Ninety percent of endoscopic diagnoses and 81% of radiological diagnoses proved to be correct.

Table 8.1 Findings in patients randomly allocated to investigation by endoscopy or radiology

	Endoscopy	Radiology
Gastric ulcer	134	83
Duodenal ulcer	122	160
Superficial erosive lesions and oesophageal ulcer	98	17
Tumours	18	13
Varices	10	5
Miscellaneous	0	2
Overall % with abnormalities	72.7	54.8

Table 8.2 Outcome in patients randomly allocated to endoscopic or radiological investigation

	Endoscopy (%)	Radiology (%)
Operations	18.1	18.2
Death	8.4	7.6
Hospital stay over 7 days	43.3	44.0

Conclusions

From our results we conclude that in a community where peptic ulceration is the commonest cause of haematemesis and melaena, and where a good double contrast barium radiography service is available, the routine performance of upper gastrointestinal endoscopy does not benefit the patient. No lowering of mortality rates or change in operation rates or length of stay is observable. Although a positive diagnosis is more likely to be made, it does not seem to help the patient.

THE ROLE OF SURGERY IN MANAGING ULCER BLEEDING

There have been no controlled trials completed which might allow one to judge whether an aggressive surgical or a conservative management policy will benefit individuals with ulcer bleeding. However, we observed some time ago that patients admitted to one of the two Nottingham hospitals with ulcer bleeding were more likely to be operated upon than if they were admitted to the other, and this difference was investigated in detail [2].

Method

Patients with haematemesis and melaena are admitted on a rota basis according to the day of the week to either of the two Nottingham Hospitals, one being on call twice as often as the other, and both having the same standard facilities. The outcome in a consecutive series of patients with gastric or duodenal ulcer bleeding was therefore investigated.

Results

Between 1977 and 1979 302 gastric and duodenal ulcer patients were admitted, 206 to hospital A and 96 to hospital B. Patients proved comparable in terms of average age, the ratio of duodenal to gastric ulcers and the severity of bleeding as judged by the lowest recorded haemoglobin concentrations (Table 8.3).

Patients were more likely to be operated upon if admitted to hospital B and

Table 8.3 Comparability of patients admitted to the two Nottingham hospitals with peptic ulcer bleeding

	Hospital A	Hospital B
No. of patients	206	96
Mean age	61.9	63.6
Ratio DU:GU	1.45	1.46
Mean lowest Hb ($\pm$ SD)	8.7 $\pm$ 2.9	8.7 $\pm$ 2.3

DU – duodenal ulcer
GU – gastric ulcer
Hb – haemoglobin concentration

Table 8.4 Frequency of operation for bleeding peptic ulcer in the Nottingham hospitals

	Hospital A	Hospital B
Operations	66 (32%)*	44 (46%)*
Timing day 0–1	26%	34%
Outcome: deaths	12.7%	17.7%

* Difference statistically significant, $P = 0.03$

operations were also slightly more likely to be carried out within the first 24 hours following admission, the difference in operation rates being statistically significant ($P = 0.03$), and probably clinically important too, patients being about 30% more likely to be operated upon at hospital B compared with hospital A (Table 8.4).

Examination of overall mortality rates showed, however, that the death rate tended to be higher in patients admitted to the hospital with the more aggressive surgical policy. This overall difference was in part due to there being more patients with severe coincidental disease of other systems being admitted to hospital B, and if this difference was taken into account the overall death rates at the two hospitals probably did not differ materially.

Examination of death rates by age shows, as might be expected, that elderly patients have high mortality rates. In general terms if a patient with a bleeding gastric or duodenal ulcer is over 65 and has an operation then the chances of death in the postoperative period are about one in four. Such deaths arise from the complications of operation and from intercurrent illness notably cardiorespiratory disease. Increasing awareness of the frequency of these sequelae has been associated in Nottingham with a fall in the frequency of operative intervention in patients with haematemesis and melaena without any rise, or even a fall in overall mortality rates. Table 8.5 compares the operation rates in 1975–77 and in 1978–80 in the Nottingham Hospitals in 908 patients with bleeding gastric and duodenal ulcers. During the period under review operation rates fell substantially so that just

Table 8.5 Outcome in bleeding peptic ulceration in Nottingham 1975–80

	Operation	Total	% operation	Overall % deaths
Gastric ulcer				
1975–1977	58	173	33.5	13.9
1978–1980	48	225	21.3	12.9
Duodenal ulcer				
1975–1977	82	244	33.6	9.4
1978–1980	57	266	21.4	9.8

over a fifth rather than a third of patients were being operated upon [3]. Mortality rates changed very little or even fell. The severity of bleeding, as judged by transfusion requirements, was unchanged suggesting that the results cannot be accounted for by a changed patient population and less severe cases being admitted in late years. The importance of timing of operation is now undergoing examination in a controlled study in Birmingham, where, so far, the tendency has been for there to be more deaths in the late operation group, although the total number of deaths so far recorded (six) is too few to allow clear judgement [4].

Assessment of the value of treatments for gastrointestinal bleeding has been bedevilled by the problem of devising and completing studies in which very large numbers of patients are included: few studies are of adequate size and few investigations realize the true extent of the problem which has exercised the minds of those treating myocardial infarction for some years [5].

Conclusion

The management of bleeding peptic ulcer in the elderly by operation may have been over-emphasised.

ACKNOWLEDGEMENTS

These studies would not have been possible without the ready cooperation of the Nottingham Hospitals' physicians and surgeons. Support from the Department of Health and Social Security is gratefully acknowledged.

REFERENCES

1. Dronfield, M. W., McIllmurray, M. B., Ferguson, R., Atkinson, M. and Langman, M. J. S. (1977) A prospective randomised study of endoscopy and radiology in acute upper gastro-intestinal tract bleeding. *Lancet*, **i**, 1167.

2. Dronfield, M. W., Atkinson, M. and Langman, M. J. S. (1979) Effect of different operation policies on mortality from bleeding peptic ulcer. *Lancet*, **i**, 1126.
3. Vellacott, K. D., Dronfield, M. W., Atkinson, M. and Langman, M. J. S. (1982) Comparison of medical and surgical management of bleeding peptic ulcers. *Br. Med. J.*, **284**, 548–50.
4. Morris, D. L., Hawker, P. C., Simms, M. H., Dykes, P. W. and Keighley, M. R. B. (1982) Optimal timing of surgery for peptic ulcer haemorrhage. *Gut*, **22**, A888.
5. Langman, M. J. S. (1981) Clinical trials in acute upper gastrointestinal bleeding. *Acta Endoscop.*, **11**, 183.

9

Upper gastrointestinal lesions

D. G. COLIN-JONES

Vascular abnormalities of the upper gastrointestinal tract have been reported sporadically for many years, but the availability of endoscopy has been responsible for a recent surge in reports which make it clear that vascular abnormalities are more common than originally supposed. The majority of reports referred to lesions in the proximal colon, but the stomach has been incriminated in several recent studies.

CLASSIFICATION AND NOMENCLATURE

There is a multiplicity of names in the literature which refer to the range of vascular malformations. Table 9.1 gives some of the more common ones. Because of the confusion two terms have been suggested as generic names – mucosal vascular abnormality (MVA) by Rogers [1] and telangiopathy by Farup *et al.* [2]. Both are open to criticism. Although the lesion is a problem because it bleeds from its mucosal surface, the vascular abnormality often extends below the mucosa. The term telangiopathy suggests a relationship to hereditary haemorrhagic telangiectasis (HHT), or Rendu–Osler–Weber syndrome, which is not always the case. The situation is made more difficult by the general acceptance of the term angiodysplasia for lesions of the proximal colon. For the purpose of this chapter the term mucosal vascular abnormality (MVA) will be used, as it appears to the author to be the most suitable term.

There is a spectrum of vascular abnormalities ranging from a cluster of abnormal vessels to true vascular neoplasms. The classification relevant to this review comes from Bongiovi and Duffy [3] (Table 9.2) and is discussed by Farup *et al.* [2] – all true neoplasms have been excluded from this survey.

Table 9.1 Nomenclature

Arteriovenous malformations
Angiodysplasia
Telangiectasia
Vascular hamartoma
Haemangioma
Aneurysmal dilatation
Vascular dilatation
Vascular ectasias
Mucosal vascular abnormality
Telangiopathy

Table 9.2 Mucosal vascular abnormalities

Haemangioma	Capillary
	Cavernous
	Mixed
Telangiectasia	Hereditary (HHT)
	Non-hereditary
	Localized
	Diffuse

Adapted from Bongiovi and Duffy, 1967 [3].

Is there a difference between the lesion of, say HHT and angiodysplasia associated with the aortic valve disease? Weaver *et al.* [4] propose a spectrum of the vascular lesions from true hereditary (HHT) through angiodysplasis to radiation (Table 9.3). They consider that the lesion of angiodysplasia contains smaller vessels more closely packed than the vessels of HHT. The difference is slight and this is confirmed by perfusion of the vascular abnormality in angio-dysplasia [5] and in HHT (Dr P. Salmon, personal communication). The lesions in hereditary and non-hereditary telangiectasis are therefore very similar and the term MVA will be used. Haemangiomas displace adjacent tissues and have vessels of different size (small – capillary, hugely dilated – cavernous). They may be only slightly elevated or polypoid. These MVA are almost certainly distinct from Dieulafoy's disease, which is an arterial malformation, usually in the fundus of the stomach and present with massive bleeding [6].

THE OESOPHAGUS

The oesophagus may be the site of telangiectases in HHT but they are much less common than further down the gut [7] where the whole length of the intestine may be affected.

The oesophagus may be the site of haemangiomas [8]. Two-thirds of benign

Table 9.3 Spectrum of vascular abnormality after Weaver *et al.*, 1979 [4]

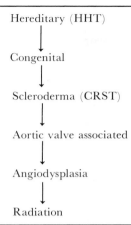

Hereditary (HHT)

↓

Congenital

↓

Scleroderma (CRST)

↓

Aortic valve associated

↓

Angiodysplasia

↓

Radiation

oesophageal tumours are leiomyomas and haemangiomas are rare – about 2% of all benign tumours in Foster's review [8]. Only 27 cases had been reported up to 1979. Two cases are presented to illustrate the problem.

CASE 1. A 75-year-old lady presented with melaena and a short dyspeptic history. There were no oesophageal symptoms. Endoscopy showed a bluish lesion in the midoesophagus, raised and soft – clearly vascular. No biopsy was taken but the appearance suggested a cavernous haemangioma. The patient had a benign gastric ulcer which was the probable source of bleeding. The haemangioma was left alone as it had not bled.

CASE 2. A 58-year-old lady presented with a haematemesis. At endoscopy a polyp was found in the lower oesophagus, about 6 mm across and 10 mm long; it was actively bleeding. Three days later, after resuscitation, the polyp was removed by diathermy snare (coagulating current). The lesion proved to be a haemangioma. Repeat endoscopy two weeks later showed complete healing with no sign of a vascular lesion.

Suspected vascular lesions of the oesophagus should *not* be biopsied (the result of biopsy in Foster's case [8] was dramatic). The use of closed forceps to check on suppleness is often helpful. Diathermy is not without risk especially in the oesophagus. The successful outcome here was due to a suitable length of stalk.

STOMACH

Diffuse antral vascular abnormalities (Fig. 9.1)

In 1978, Lewis *et al.* [9] reported a patient with diffuse streaking red erythematous vascular lesions in the antrum who was experiencing recurrent anaemia.

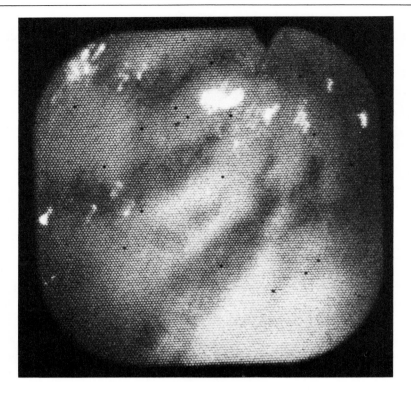

Fig. 9.1 Antral mucosal vascular abnormality. Linear streaks of dilated vessels superficial in the mucosa are seen radiating from the vicinity of the pylorus.

Histologically the vessels were dilated and tortuous. Subsequently this report was confirmed by three more cases [10] one of whom was losing up to 200 ml of blood per day. One patient died (she was 79 and frail) but in the remaining cases partial gastrectomy was curative. More recently [11] an identical lesion in the antrum was found to be responsible for recurrent anaemia over a 15-year period. This patient appeared to stop bleeding when steroids were given (prednisolone 30 mg daily at first). This observation needs confirmation.

The author has had two such cases also presenting with recurrent anaemia, one of whom was cured by partial gastrectomy (which removed the lesion). The lesions were on the folds of the antrum, radiating in a stellate manner from near the pylorus with a fine nodular appearance on close inspection. These red nodular and tortuous vessels blanched on pressure from closed forceps. In none of the cases reported (including this one) have biopsies resulted in dramatic blood loss or diagnostic abnormality in the samples, but dilated submucosal vessels were a feature. In the second case, an elderly female, cure of the recurrent bleeding and near elimination of the visible vascular abnormality was achieved by multiple injections of sclerosant over a period of four months (using sodium tetradecyl sulphate, 0.5 ml at each injection, 12–15 ml being used at each of five sessions).

Localized mucosal vascular abnormalities (Fig. 9.2)

Recent reports have highlighted the importance of these lesions [2, 4, 12, 13] which may arise either *de novo* or in association with other conditions. Associations have been with aortic valve disease, especially aortic stenosis [1, 4] radiation to the abdomen [4] scleroderma (CRST-calcinosis, Raynaud's sclerodactyly and telangiectasis) and Von Willebrand's disease [4, 15]. Their frequency may be as high as 1 in 285 cases of routine upper gastrointestinal endoscopy [12]. Most patients have been elderly.

There are, of course, many reports of vascular lesions associated with HHT [4, 16, 17, 18]. These lesions may be single or multiple and there are usually important clues in the forms of skin lesions, epitaxis or a family history.

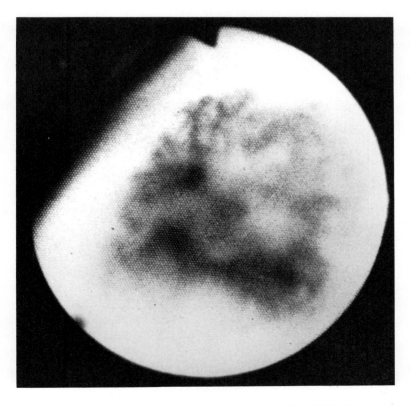

Fig.9.2 Close-up view of solitary mucosal vascular abnormality which is approximately 3 mm across. Fine blood vessels can be seen as dark lines against a paler background.

Personal series of non-HHT cases of vascular malformations

Six cases (three male, three female) have been seen in the last two years with an average age of 76 years. One patient had aortic valve disease and additional lesions in the ascending colon. Another (now aged 83) had two such lesions in the stomach and multiple lesions in the small and large intestines: no therapy, which has included electrocoagulation, vagotomy, right hemicolectomy and ligation of lesions at laparotomy, has given lasting control of recurrent bleeding.

The lesions have chiefly been located in the fundus or body of the stomach (one in the antrum). These have been discrete, about 4–6 mm across with a pale halo around a bright red dot. Close inspection showed multiple fine vessels spreading out 1 mm or so from the central slightly elevated bleb. In the two cases seen soon after a bleed a small dark breach in the mucosa could be seen in the centre.

All patients were treated with monopolar electrocoagulation (Fig. 9.3). This was accompanied by bleeding which it was always possible to control by further coagulation. Follow-up one week later revealed an ulcer with MVA at the edge of the diathermy ulcer (two patients), huge vessels in the base of the induced ulcer (three patients) and obliteration of the lesion (one patient). Four patients had one repeat diathermy and one patient two further treatments. Despite the disturbing size of the vessels in the base of the postdiathermy ulcer, healing occurred (with scarring) in about three weeks without visible vessels. All five patients were cured of their bleeding.

This personal experience is very similar to that reported by Weaver [4] who advised delaying for at least a week between coagulations – advice with which I concur.

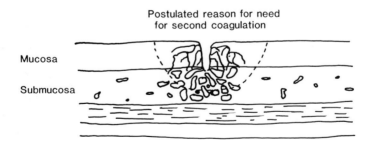

Fig. 9.3 It is suggested that the blood vessels which bleed are superficial in the mucosa, but that there are other blood vessels deeper in the submucosa which are not coagulated by the first diathermy coagulation. The dotted line represents the area which is diathermied. Some blood vessels may not be coagulated if they are deep to this area of tissue destruction.

Other treatments have been embolization of bleeding vessels using selective catheterization [13], resection of the affected part of the gut after detailed investigation [19] and in some centres laser photocoagulation [20].

Gastric haemangiomas

These are very rare [2]. In 1967 Bongiovi and Duffy [3] found only 35 previously reported cases and the number is probably still less than 50. It would appear that they are often polypoid and present with blood loss.

DUODENAL MUCOSAL VASCULAR ABNORMALITIES

MVA are usually found in the duodenum as part of HHT [16, 17] but may occasionally occur in non-hereditary cases [2, 4, 7]. They have the same appearances as MVA elsewhere in the gastrointestinal tract. Especially in HHT the whole length of the small gut may be affected, but even in isolated, non-hereditary cases the duodenum distal to the cap may be the site of MVA. Furthermore bleeding through the papilla from the biliary or pancreatic duct may be important (see CASE 3 below). It is therefore essential to inspect the second part of the duodenum at endoscopy for upper gastrointestinal bleeding when no cause has been established proximal to the cap. This is illustrated by the following case report.

CASE 3. A man aged 65 presented with recurrent anaemia. At his first endoscopy a blood streak in the distal duodenum was attributed to endoscopic trauma. Three months later after a recurrence of anaemia (Hb 5.6 g), the same streak was noted. This time a more careful check was made and blood found oozing from the papilla. Detailed investigation showed a daily blood loss of about 30 ml day^{-1}. Endoscopic retrograde pancreatography (ERCP) and arteriograms were unhelpful. Eventually the lesion was found to be an MVA of the pancreatic duct at the junction of the main and accessory ducts which was successfully coagulated at laparotomy (Professor L. Blumgart).

CONCLUSION

MVA of the upper gastrointestinal tract are being increasingly recognized in the non-hereditary form. They are often found in the elderly patient. In the stomach endoscopic control by electro- or photocoagulation seems to be the treatment of choice where the lesions are few. The lesions are small but characteristic – all endoscopists need to be on the lookout for them.

REFERENCES

1. Rogers, B. H. G. (1980) Endoscopic diagnosis and therapy of mucosal vascular abnormalities of the gastrointestinal tract occurring in elderly patients and associated with cardiac, vascular and pulmonary disease. *Gastrointest. Endosc.*, **26** (4).
2. Farup, P. G., Rosseland, A., Stray, N., Pitts, R. *et al.* (1981) Localised telangiopathy of the stomach and duodenum diagnosed and treated endoscopically. *Endoscopy*, **12**, 1–6.
3. Bongiovi, J. H. and Duffy, J. L. (1967) Gastric haemangioma associated with upper gastrointestinal bleeding. *Arch. Surg.*, **95**, 93.
4. Weaver, G. A., Alpern, H. D., Davis, J. S., Ramsey, W. H. and Reichelderfer, M. (1979) Gastrointestinal angiodysplasia associated with aortic valve disease. Part of a spectrum of angiodysplasia of the gut. *Gastroenterology*, **77**, 1–11.
5. Cohen, J. I. (1980) Angiodysplasia of the gut. *John Hopkins Med. J.*, **146**, 211–15.
6. Mortensen, N. J. M., Mountford, R. A., Davies, J. D. and Jeans, W. D. (1983) Dieulafoy's disease: a distinctive arteriovenous malformation causing massive gastric haemorrhage. *Br. J. Surg.*, **70**, 76–8.
7. Mcgee, R. R. (1979) Oestrogen-progesterone therapy for gastrointestinal bleeding in hereditary haemorrhagic telangiectasis. *South Med. J.*, **71**, 1503.
8. Foster, C. A., Yomehiro, E. G. and Benjamin, R. B. (1978) Oesophageal haemangioma. *ENT J.*, **57**, 455–9.
9. Lewis, T. D., Laufer, I. and Goodacre, R. L. (1978) Arteriovenous malformation of the stomach. *Dig. Dis.*, **23**, 467–71.
10. Wheeler, M. H., Smith, P. M., Cotton, P. B., Evans, D. M. D. and Lawrie, B. W. (1979) Abnormal blood vessels in the gastric antrum. *Dig. Dis. Sci.*, **24**, 155–8.
11. Calam, J. and Walker, R. J. (1980) Antral vascular lesion, achlorhydria and chronic gastrointestinal blood loss. *Dig. Dis. Sci.*, **25**, 236–9.
12. Blankenstein, M. Van., Dees, J. and Tenkate, F. J. W. (1978) Bleeding arteriovenous malformations diagnosed by endoscopy. *Gut*, **19** (A), 432.
13. Sherman, L., Shenoy, S. S., Neumann, P. R., Barrios, G. G. and Peer, R. M. (1979) Arteriovenous malformation of the stomach. *Am. J. Gastroenterol.*, **72**, 160–4.
14. Rosenkrans, P. C. M., de Rooy, D. J., Bosman, F. T., Eulderink, F. and Cats, A. (1980) Gastrointestinal telangiectasia as a cause of severe blood loss in systemic sclerosis. *Endoscopy*, **12**, 200–4.
15. McGrath, K. M., Johnson, C. A. and Stuart, J. J. (1979) Acquired von Willebrand disease associated with an inhibitor to factor VIII antigen and gastrointestinal telangiectasis. *Am. J. Med.*, **67**, 693–6.
16. Moore, J. D., Thompson, N. W., Appelman, H. D. and Foley, D. (1978) Arteriovenous malformations of the gastrointestinal tract. *Arch. Surg.*, **111**, 381–9.
17. Posner, D. E. and Sampliner, R. E. (1978) Hereditary haemorrhagic telangiectasis in three black men. *Am. J. Gastroenterol.*, **70**, 389–92.
18. Ona, F. V. and Ahluwalia, M. (1980) Endoscopic appearances of gastric angiodysplasia in hereditary haemorrhagic telangiectasis. *Am. J. Gastroenterol.*, **73**, 148–9.
19. Owen, W. J. (1979) Hereditary haemorrhagic telangiectasis. Major recurrent gastric bleeding treated by gastrectomy. *J. R. Soc. Med.*, **72**, 937–9.
20. Jensen, D. M., Machicado, G., Tapia, J., Mautner, W. and Franco, P. (1980) Endoscopic treatment of telangiectasis with argon laser photocoagulation. *Abstr. Am. Soc. Gastrointest. Endosc.*, **May**.
21. Bourdette, D. and Greenberg, B. (1979) Twelve year history of gastrointestinal bleeding in a patient with calcific aortic stenosis and haemorrhagic telangiectasis. *Dig. Dis. Sci.*, **24**, 77–9.

IO

Angiodysplasia of the colon

RICHARD H. HUNT

INTRODUCTION

Vascular abnormalities of the colon are a well recognized although relatively uncommon cause of bleeding from the gastrointestinal tract [1, 2, 3]. The first recorded vascular abnormality causing bleeding from the large bowel was reported by Phillips in 1839 [4], who described an erectile tumour of the anus. Despite this early report few series of patients with gastrointestinal bleeding have mentioned vascular abnormalities as a cause of haemorrhage until recent years. Not surprisingly there has been confusion within the literature where most workers have tended to use the term angioma and angiodysplasia synonomously [5, 6, 7, 8, 9] while all emphasize the diagnostic difficulties which these lesions cause in clinical practice. In 1963 Catem and Jiminez [10] suggested that as many as 27% of patients with a vascular abnormality may go undiagnosed but once a lesion has been identified either radiologically or endoscopically and its exact anatomical location and extent is known the management may be relatively easy.

In recent years there has been considerable interest in those vascular abnormalities which affect the caecum and right colon. Boley and his colleagues [11] have clarified the nature of these lesions and defined those which have usually been referred to as angiodysplasia as degenerative in origin. In contrast those lesions which are hamartomatous in origin should probably best be described as angiomas [12].

Lesions have been particularly recognized by radiologists since the initial report by Margulis and colleagues in 1960 [13] who identified a vascular malformation in the caecum of a 60-year-old lady, who presented with massive bleeding. Numerous reports followed the introduction of selective mesenteric angiography when the characteristic radiographic features can be more readily observed.

Since colonoscopy has been more widely practised and proved of such value in the diagnosis of patients with unexplained rectal bleeding [12, 14–16], the lesions of angiodysplasia have been more frequently recognized at endoscopy [7–9, 17–21]. Colonoscopy has the advantage that these lesions may be successfully treated at the time of the diagnostic procedure using the diathermy coagulation forceps developed by Williams [22] [7, 18, 20, 23].

AETIOLOGY AND PATHOLOGY

The lesions of angiodysplasia commonly occur in the caecum and ascending colon and some workers believe that the lesions only occur at these sites [11] while others have reported similar lesions in the stomach [20, 24–26] and elsewhere in the colon [27].

Boley and his colleagues [11] suggest that those lesions occurring in the caecum and right colon represent a separate and unique entity from previously described vascular lesions of the gastrointestinal tract. These conclusions are based on the results of their elegant injection techniques and a meticulous study of the histopathology of the lesions. Baum and his colleagues [28] suggested that these are acquired lesions attributable to mucosal ischaemia, resulting from arteriovenous shunting in the mucosa, which occurs with changes in intracolonic pressure. In contrast Boley et al. [11] explain the development of the lesion by chronic intermittent partial obstruction of the submucosal veins where they traverse the longitudinal and circular muscle layers of the bowel. Occurring repeatedly over many years, this occlusion of the low pressure veins, does not affect the higher pressure arterial inflow. This pressure differential results in capillary vessel dilatation, capillary ring dilatation and loss of competence of the precapillary sphincters which creates small arteriovenous malformations at the level of the mucosal capillaries. The frequency with which this lesion is observed in the right colon is attributed to Laplace's law. When applied to the colon this suggests that the tension in the muscles of the bowel wall will be greater in that part of the colon with the greatest diameter, which is the caecum [29]. Boley and his colleagues [11] suggested that if angiodysplasia were due to aging it should be present in elderly patients who have not yet bled from a lesion. In order to test this hypothesis they studied a control group of 15 colons and identified mucosal ectasias in 27% and a large dilated submucosal vein in 53%.

Galloway et al. [30] who noted an association with aortic stenosis suggested that the lesions developed as a consequence of decreased perfusion pressure secondary to a decreased left ventricular output. Rogers [20] whose patients were all diagnosed at colonoscopy, noted an association with both aortic valve disease and chronic lung disease, and he has suggested that lowered oxygen tension in the end arterial supply of the superior mesenteric vessels results in capillary dilatation and proliferation and eventually a true vascular abnormality. In contrast Weaver and his colleagues [26] have suggested that vascular ectasias of the gastrointestinal tract represent a spectrum with inherited lesions such as Rendu–Osler–Weber disease at one end of the spectrum and acquired lesions at the other; these workers describe lesions similar to angiodysplasia occurring in the stomach as well as in the colon.

Although in many series 20–25% of patients including those reported by Boley *et al.* [11] have aortic valve disease they do not believe that this condition contributes to the development of mucosal ectasias although low perfusion pressure, and hypoxia may cause ischaemic necrosis of the single layer of endothelium which separates the vessel from the colonic lumen (Fig. 10.1).

The pathology of angiodysplasia of the colon has been described in detail by Mitsudo *et al* [31] who have demonstrated a spectrum from early small focal lesions to multiple large advanced lesions. Under light microscopy early lesions show tortuous, dilated submucosal veins. These communicate with the superficial mucosal capillaries which may or may not be dilated, and mildly compress the lamina propria. In the later stages of the condition the changes in the submucosa are more apparent and there is marked ectasia of mucosal vessels. The submucosal veins become very dilated and tortuous while the arteries are normal (Fig. 10.1).

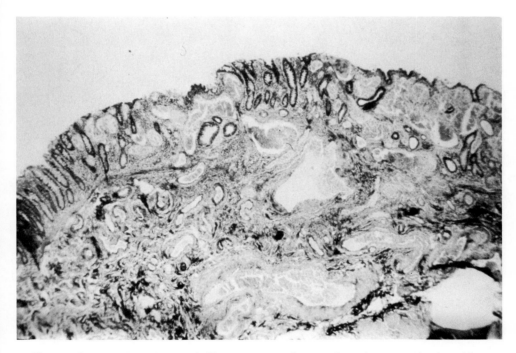

Fig. 10.1 Gross specimen (× 21.25). Shows tortuous submucosal vessels communicating with two areas of mucosal angiodysplasia (upper R and upper L). A platelet thrombus plugs the site of haemorrhage (upper R) and is seen again in Fig. 10.4.

These communicate with the mucosal capillaries which are continuous with small or large groups of dilated vessels which compress the crypts. In the advanced lesions the attenuated epithelium and capillary wall is all that separates the capillary lumen from the colonic lumen (Figs 10.2 and 10.3). It is clear from these examples how easily the wall may rupture and result in colonic haemorrhage. The site of a platelet plug and organizing thrombus extending into the colonic lumen after an episode of bleeding is seen in Fig. 10.4.

CLINICAL PRESENTATION

The vascular lesions which most commonly affect the colon occur in the older age groups and all series report a mean age of 60–70 years [11, 19, 27, 28, 32–36] and an almost equal sex incidence. The majority of patients have experienced one or more episodes of rectal bleeding varying from massive haemorrhage and cardiovascular shock to slow occult blood loss presenting only as anaemia. The pattern of bleeding varies both between and within individuals, but even when severe is usually self limiting. Bleeding is more frequently bright red but maroon coloured or tarry stools may occur. Characteristically patients have had one or

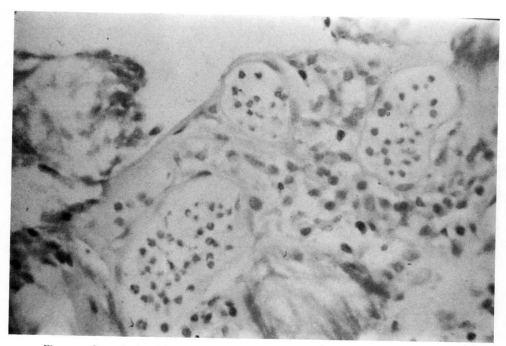

Fig. 10.2 Coagulation biopsy specimen (× 340). Dilated ectatic thin walled superficial capillaries with effete red cells in the vessels.

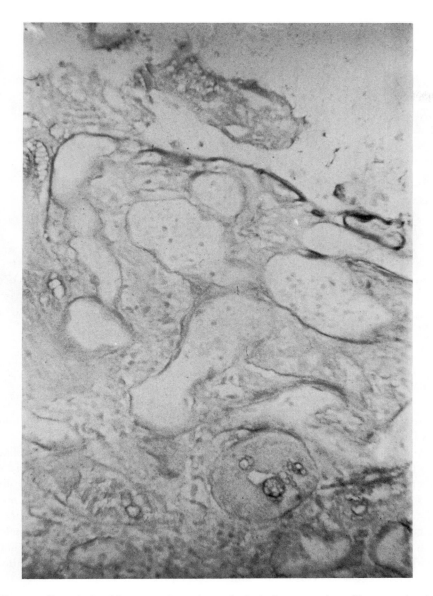

Fig. 10.3 Coagulation biopsy specimen ($\times$ 250). A similar example to Fig. 10.2 showing distortion of the superficial capillaries and the thin vessel wall adjacent to the colonic lumen with no protective overlying mucosa.

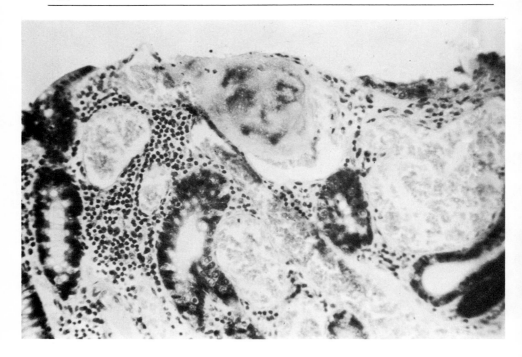

Fig. 10.4 Gross specimen (× 212.5). Large ectatic superficial capillaries with platelet plug and organizing thrombus (at the centre) at the site of capillary rupture.

more operations for diagnosis such as duodenal ulcer or diverticular disease, which has been considered the source of blood loss.

An association between aortic stenosis and obscure gastrointestinal bleeding was first noted by Heyde [37] and again by Williams [38]. This and a variety of other conditions have been reported in most recent series and were clinically evident in up to 80% of patients in one series [20]. Aortic stenosis is still the most commonly reported lesion [7, 20, 26, 39] although few cases have been confirmed by catheterization. Aortic sclerosis may also occur and hypertension, atherosclerosis and other vascular disease constitute the remainder of the cardiovascular conditions. An association with Von Willebrand's disease and gastrointestinal bleeding due to a vascular abnormality has been recognized [40–42] but it is not clear how closely the pathology of the associated vascular lesion correlates with that of true angiodysplasia as described by Mitsudo *et al.* [31].

DIAGNOSIS

Until recent years the lesions of angiodysplasia have been diagnosed most successfully by radiological techniques especially since the development of selective mesenteric angiography [28, 32, 43–45]. The subsequent improvements in diagnostic methods using subtraction films has enabled the radiologist to define a number of important radiological criteria for diagnosis (Table 10.1). These include particularly a vascular tuft, which represents the capillary network, an early filling vein and a dense slowly emptying vein [46]. These major features may be present alone or in combination and when present should always suggest to the radiologist the possibility of a vascular abnormality. When extravasation of contrast media is seen in association with the above criteria active bleeding from a ruptured angiodysplasia is probable but if the typical features are not present bleeding from a vascular ectasia is unlikely [46].

The first reports of angiodysplasia observed at colonoscopy were by Skibba *et al.* [8] and Rogers and Adler [7] and these are now recognized as an important cause of colonic haemorrhage which should be exhaustively sought by the colonoscopist. The typical endoscopic appearance of angiodysplasia includes a cherry red lesion seldom more than 5 mm in size with a slightly raised dilated central vessel under tension and with radiating peripheral vessels (Figs 10.5 and 10.6).

Diagnosis may also be made at operation when angiodysplasia can often be seen on careful examination of the mucosal surface immediately after resection of a segment of the colon [47]. No obvious changes of angiodysplasia are seen on the serosal surface of the colon at surgery although abnormalities may be seen with angiomatous lesions. This distinction emphasizes the importance of delineating the extent of the angiodysplasia lesion by colonoscopy or angiography or both prior to surgery. In patients who are suspected to have a vascular malformation peroperative colonoscopy of the large or small bowel may be especially helpful to transilluminate the bowel wall. The surgeon views from the serosal aspect, pleating segments of bowel over the colonoscope, which is passed under direct view by the endoscopist [48, 49].

Table 10.1 Angiographic criteria of angiodysplasia

Vascular tuft
Intramucosal vein: densely opacified, tortuous, slowly emptying
Early filling vein

The diagnosis of angiodysplasia is confirmed by the histopathologist either on the resection specimen or following coagulation biopsy [50]. The histopathological criteria have been detailed earlier in this chapter under *Aetiology and pathology* (see page 98). The essential feature is the presence of dilated ectatic communicating mucosal capillaries. The combination of an endoscopically typical lesion, *in vivo* photography, and supportive histology has been a very satisfactory way of establishing the diagnosis, so much so that coagulation biopsy is probably no longer necessary if a typical lesion has been identified endoscopically [33].

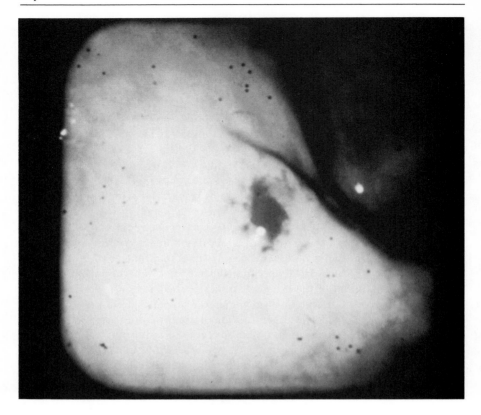

Fig. 10.5 Angiodysplasia lesion lying above the ileocaecal valve. The lesion is cherry red, the dilated central vessel is under tension with smaller radiating peripheral capillaries.

PRACTICAL EXPERIENCE

We have now had experience of 26 patients with angiodysplasia referred for colonoscopy at the Royal Naval Hospital, Haslar for recurrent bleeding per rectum or anaemia.

Methods

All patients underwent thorough bowel preparation before colonoscopy [51] which included restriction of dietary fibre, increased fluid intake and purgation followed on the day of the procedure by either tap water enemas or oral mannitol.

Colonoscopy was performed using ACM, Fuji or Olympus Instruments and diazepam and pethidine were given intravenously for sedation and analgesia as

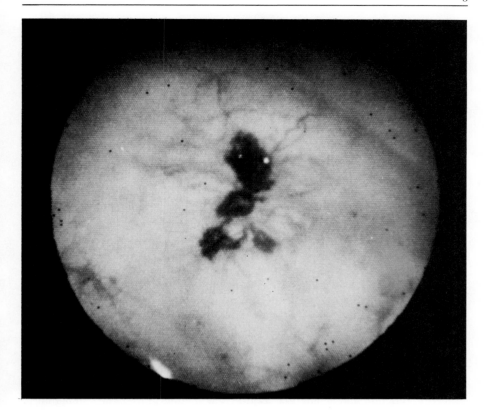

Fig. 10.6 Angiodysplasia lesion in the caecum. The lesion is bright red and the dilated irregular superficial vessels can be clearly seen.

required. The angiodysplasia lesions were photographed before coagulation was performed and coagulation was only attempted if the number of lesions visualized numbered five or less. An attempt was made for the forceps always to be placed at the periphery of the lesion. Once grasped the lesion was then pulled towards the lumen of the colon. This 'tents' the mucosa and submucosa away from the outer layers of the colonic wall which is particularly thin in the caecum increasing the risk of transmural coagulation or perforation [34]. The apex of the 'tent' is pulled asymmetrically over the centre of the abnormality to enhance coagulation in the mucosa and submucosa at the site of the angiodysplasia lesion (Fig. 10.7). Coagulation was performed at no more than 25 watts applied for very short bursts to achieve a very small and controlled superficial coagulation (Fig. 10.8). When mannitol bowel preparation had been used CO_2 was routinely insufflated before electrocoagulation was attempted because of the theoretical risk of intracolonic

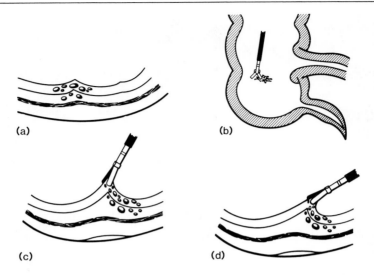

Fig. 10.7 The technique of coagulation of angiodysplasia lesions. (a) The lesion is predominantly in the mucosa and submucosa. (b) The lesion is grasped in the biopsy forceps at the periphery of the lesion. (c) The lesion is 'tented' into the lumen and pulled over itself (d) before the short burst of low power current is applied.

explosion [52]. Biopsies were then orientated on ground glass or filter paper and fixed in 10% buffered formal saline or in some instances 4% buffered glutaraldehyde for later plastic processing. Staining methods have included haematoxylin and eosin reticulin and alcian blue. Endoscopic photographs of the lesion and the histology were later collated to confirm the diagnosis.

Results

Colonoscopy has been performed in a total of 26 patients with a mean age of 69.9 years (47–85). There were nine male and 17 female patients. Sixteen patients (61.5%) presented with anaemia which was often profound (mean haemoglobin 8.0 G dl^{-1}). Twenty patients (77%) described bleeding per rectum and 14 (70%) of these reported more than five episodes of bleeding or malaena; five (25%) reported between one and five bleeds while only one patient described a single bleed. Patients presenting with melaena or anaemia alone had a lower haemoglobin (7.8 G dl) than those who reported overt rectal bleeding (11.1 G dl^{-1}). Both the number of episodes of bleeding and the number of lesions seen endoscopically were inversely related to the haemoglobin at presentation, while there was no relationship between the number of lesions seen at colonoscopy and the number of episodes of bleeding.

Many patients had concomitant pathology which included ten (38%) with hypertension and seven (27%) with ischaemic heart disease. Aortic valve disease

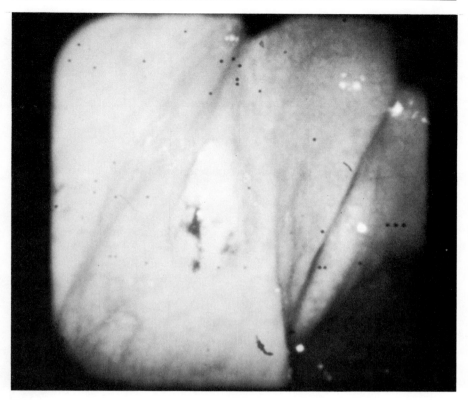

Fig. 10.8 The angiodysplasia lesion seen in Fig. 10.5 after initial coagulation. The carefully controlled and limited coagulation effect can be clearly seen. A further limited coagulation was then applied with the forceps placed at the lower pole of the lesion.

was recorded in four (15%) while two patients had thyroid disease. One patient had undergone radiotherapy to the pelvis for a previous seminoma of the right testis and one patient was discovered at the time of recurrent bleeding after surgery to have Von Willebrand's disease.

All the 26 patients had been extensively investigated before their referral to colonoscopy and had accumulated 162 negative investigations between them (Table 10.2). Two had undergone gastric surgery for a suspected peptic ulcer. Total colonoscopy was performed in all 26 patients; seven patients have had two and two patients three colonoscopies. Five repeat examinations were performed for subsequent further bleeding and four as routine follow-up examinations to see if coagulation had been effective at eliminating the lesions. Twenty patients (77%) had more than one angiodysplasia lesion seen at their initial colonoscopy, and 11 of these had more than five lesions visible. All were in the caecum and or ascending

Table 10.2 Previous negative investigations in 26 patients with angiodysplasia

Barium meal	21
Barium enema	41
Rigid sigmoidoscopy	61
Upper gastrointestinal endoscopy	38
Mesenteric angiography	1

colon and none were seen distal to the hepatic flexure. Lesions were often seen in close proximity to the ileocaecal valve.

During the 37 colonoscopies 64 individual coagulations were performed and 35 biopsies were taken, in 23 of the 26 patients. Histological confirmation was obtained in 11 patients (48%) while in a further eight histology assessed together with the endoscopist's opinion and photography strongly supported a diagnosis of angiodysplasia. The lesions were so extensive (Fig. 10.9) in the further three patients that primary surgical resection was considered to be the correct management and biopsies were not taken. Histological confirmation of the diagnosis was obtained in each of these patients following right hemicolectomy and immediate processing of the specimens.

In four patients histology did not support the diagnosis of angiodysplasia despite endoscopically and photographically typical lesions which had been documented. One of these patients suffered a delayed perforation of the caecum after coagulation when open biopsy at the time of surgical repair confirmed the diagnosis. One patient died nine months after diagnosis following a further bleed at which time post mortem revealed no angiodysplasia but extensive gastric erosions, bronchopneumonia and a carcinoma of the bronchus. In the third patient who had presented with recurrent anaemia, there was no recurrence of anaemia one year after coagulation of two caecal angiodysplasia lesions.

Follow-up

A questionnaire was mailed to all referring consultants in June 1981 seeking follow up details of all patients including any episodes of further bleeding and surgical intervention. The mean period of follow-up was 17 months (range 2–36 months).

Eleven (46%) of the 26 patients had suffered further bleeding at some time after their initial colonoscopy. Six of these patients had further angiodysplasia lesions at repeat colonoscopy which had either been missed at the initial examination or were new lesions which had developed in the interim. Two further patients were presumed by their clinicians to have bled again from angiodysplasia and endoscopy was not requested, while the remaining patients were bleeding from the upper gastrointestinal tract in two cases and from haemorrhoids in one case.

Right hemicolectomy was performed after diagnosis in five patients and after rebleeding in a further two. In one patient who also had a sigmoid carcinoma a

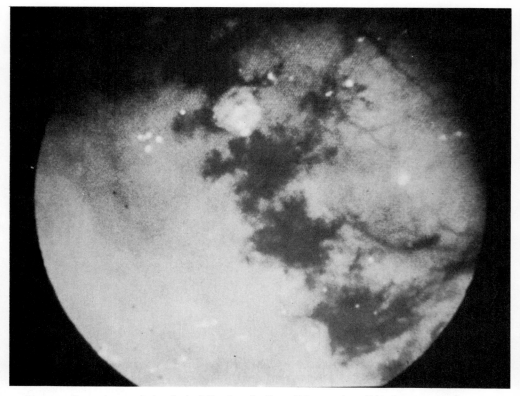

Fig. 10.9 Extensive angiodysplasia following the line of the taenia coli in the caecum. An area of ulceration can be seen in the upper part of the field of view. This patient was referred for right hemicolectomy.

local resection of the tumour was performed in addition. Repeat colonoscopy was performed at a variable interval after initial diagnosis and coagulation in four patients who had reported no further bleeding to see if there had been any recurrence of lesions. In three patients the examination was entirely normal but in the fourth a further small lesion was seen high in the caecum and this was successfully coagulated.

Discussion

The lesion of angiodysplasia has created great interest amongst clinicians, radiologists, endoscopists and pathologists and is now appreciated as an important cause of gastrointestinal bleeding. Most series report an increasing frequency in patients in their sixties and seventies [11, 19, 20, 53] which has also been our own experience [33] although angiodysplasia has been reported in patients as young as 18 [19, 54].

If a vascular abnormality is suspected as a possible diagnosis it is important to examine the patient carefully for aortic valve disease, Rendu–Osler–Weber lesions, etc. and if angiodysplasia is found Von Willebrand's disease should also be excluded.

At colonoscopy a meticulous examination of the colon and especially the caecum must be made after the best possible bowel preparation if these small lesions are not to be missed. Oral mannitol has been found an especially good preparation for cleansing the right colon but CO_2 should always be used before electrocoagulation because of the theoretical risk of a gas explosion [52]. Because of the frequency of lesions close to the ileocaecal valve it is wise to invert the colonoscope in the caecum to visualize the inferior aspect of the valve.

Although lesions described as angiodysplasia have been reported in the stomach [20, 24–26] and elsewhere in the colon [27] the distribution of angiodysplasia in our series was in keeping with the experience reported by Boley and his colleagues [11] with all the lesions in the caecum and ascending colon. One possible lesion from the sigmoid region had none of the typical histological appearances that we saw in the other coagulation biopsies or in the more extensive resection specimens. All our histology was similar to that described by Mitsudo et al. [31] showing dilated ectatic superficial mucosal vessels, compressing the crypts and sometimes associated with larger submucosal veins draining the lesion.

Although there is one report of angiodysplasia treated by angiographic embolization [55], diagnosis by angiography invariably requires further intervention by surgery to treat this condition which has meant 2 invasive procedures being performed in elderly patients with the increased risk of morbidity or mortality. A surgical mortality of 2.6% was reported by Richardson et al. [56] in their series of 39 patients with vascular abnormalities of the gastrointestinal tract. Colonoscopy offers the advantage of diagnosis combined with treatment by electrocoagulation providing that the lesions are accessible and not numerous. In our experience lesions between 5 mm and 10 mm in size can safely be treated by electrocoagulation. Haemorrhage occurred during one coagulation when the forceps were closed across the centre of the lesion. In this case the haemorrhage was relatively easily controlled at the time of endoscopy by flushing the lesion with iced water containing adrenalin (5 ml 1:1000 per 50 ml water). It is advisable however to try and pick the lesion up at the periphery repeating the procedure at the opposite quadrant if complete coagulation is not obtained initially (Fig. 10.7). Delayed perforation occurred in one patient at about 72 hours after the procedure and at the time of colonoscopy it was considered by the endoscopist that too long a coagulation had been applied. This patient had undergone cholecystectomy some years previously and at operation for the perforation it was noted that the omentum was fixed and had not covered the site of perforation. Previous abdominal surgery should perhaps be considered a relative contraindication to electrocoagulation in the caecum which is thin walled and at greater risk of transmural coagulation or frank perforation.

Electrocoagulation at colonoscopy was used without morbidity or mortality in the 27 patients reported by Rogers [20] who considered biopsy at the time of coagulation most important to differentiate the lesions from traumatic ecchymoses. In our opinion the experienced colonoscopist can readily recognize the variations of angiodysplasia and he should meticulously examine each segment of colon and the caecum before intubating it or manipulating the instrument with the attendant risk of mucosal trauma.

We believe that biopsy is unnecessary and that this will increase the margin of safety of the procedure [33] and perforation will be less of a hazard. Although the lesions diagnosed at colonoscopy are probably early lesions pathology of gross specimens by conventional and especially injection techniques confirms large underlying submucosal vessels. These larger veins may constitute a hazard to local electrocoagulation especially if a biopsy is undertaken exposing an incompletely coagulated vein.

SUMMARY AND CONCLUSION

Bleeding per rectum is a common clinical problem which may cause considerable problems in diagnosis. A combined approach between gastroenterologist/endoscopist/radiologist/surgeon and histopathologist can lead to earlier more accurate diagnosis by choosing the most appropriate initial investigations and their order. Angiodysplasia should be considered as a possible cause of bleeding especially when conventional diagnostic methods have proved negative. Colonoscopy has proved an accurate and safe technique for the diagnosis of angiodysplasia and electrocoagulation and biopsy can provide a safe treatment and confirmed histological diagnosis although the need for confirmatory biopsy has already been questioned. The colonoscopic approach is well tolerated and safer than primary surgery except for those patients with extensive lesions who will require a resection. Further carefully performed clinical and histopathological studies are required to clarify the controversy over the exact aetiology and anatomical site of these lesions.

ACKNOWLEDGEMENTS

I should like to thank my colleagues Oliver Howard for his help with the data on our 26 patients and John Buchanan for his painstaking work with the histopathology material and the departments of Clinical Illustration and Photography for their help.

REFERENCES

1. Allred, H. W. and Spencer, R. J. (1974) Hemangiomas of the colon, rectum and anus. *Mayo Clin. Proc.*, **49**, 739–41.

2. Gentry, R. W., Dockerty, M. B. and Clagett, O. T. (1949) Vascular malformations and vascular tumours of the gastrointestinal tract. *Int. Abstr. Surg.*, **88**, 281–323.

3. Shepherd, J. A. (1953) Angiomatous conditions of the gastrointestinal tract. *Br. J. Surg.*, **40**, (163), 409–21.

4. Phillips, B. (1839) Surgical cases. *Lond. Med. Gaz.*, **23**, 514–17.

5. Bartelheimer, W., Remmele, W. and Ottenjann, R. (1972) Colonoscopic recognition of hemangiomas in the colon ascendens. *Endoscopy*, **4**, 109–14.

6. Richardson, J. D., McInnis, W. D., Ramos, R. and Aust. J. B. (1975) Occult gastrointestinal bleeding: an evaluation of available diagnostic methods. *Arch. Surg.*, **110**, 661–5.

7. Rogers, B. H. G. and Adler, F. (1976) Haemangiomas of the caecum. *Gastroenterology*, **71**, 1079–82.

8. Skibba, R. M., Hartong, W. A., Mantz, F. A., Hinthorn, D. R. and Rhodes, J. B. (1976) Angiodysplasia of the caecum: colonoscopic diagnosis. *Gastrointest. Endosc.*, **22**, 177–9.

9. Wolff, W. I., Grossman, M. G. and Shinya, H. (1977) Angiodysplasia of the colon: diagnosis and treatment. *Gastroenterology*, **72**, 329–33.

10. Catem, W. S. and Jiminez, F. A. (1963) Vascular malformations of the intestine: their role as a source of haemorrhage. *Arch. Surg.*, **86**, 571–9.

11. Boley, S. J., Sammartano, R., Adamas, A., DiBiase, A. *et al.* (1977) On the nature and aetiology of vascular ectasias of the colon: degenerative lesions of ageing. *Gastroenterology*, **72**, 650–60.

12. Hunt, R. H. (1978) Rectal bleeding. *Clin. Gastroenterol.*, **7**, 719–40.

13. Margulis, A. R., Heinbecker, P. and Bernard, H. R. (1960) Operative mesenteric arteriography in the search for the site of bleeding in unexplained gastrointestinal bleeding. *Surgery*, **48**, 534–9.

14. Hunt, R. H., Swarbrick, E. T., Teague, R. H., Thomas, B. M. *et al.* (1979) Colonoscopy for unexplained rectal bleeding. *Gastroenterology*, **76**, 1158.

15. Swarbrick, E. T. and Hunt, R. H. (1981) in *Colonoscopy, Techniques, Clinical Practice and Colour Atlas*, (eds R. H. Hunt and J. D. Waye), Chapman and Hall, London, pp. 267–88.

16. Waye, J. D. (1976) Colonoscopy in rectal bleeding. *South Afr. J. Surg.*, **14**, 143–9.

17. Howard, O. M., Buchanan, J. D. and Hunt, R. H. (1981) Angiodysplasia (letter). *Lancet*, **ii**, 1340.

18. Hunt, R. H. (1980) Colonoscopy in the diagnosis and management of angiodysplasia. *Abstr. IV Eur. Congr. Gastrointest. Endosc.*, **E26**, (1), 97.

19. Max, M. H., Richardson, J. D., Flint, L. M., Knutson, C. O. and Schwesinger, W. (1981) Colonoscopic diagnosis of angiodysplasias of the gastrointestinal tract. *Surg. Gynaecol. Obstet.*, **152**, 195–9.

20. Rogers, B. H. G. (1980) Endoscopic diagnosis and therapy of mucosal vascular abnormality of the gastrointestinal tract occurring in elderly patients and associated with cardiac, vascular and pulmonary disease. *Gastrointest. Endosc.*, **26**, 134–8.

21. Swarbrick, E. T., Fevre, D. I., Hunt, R. H., Thomas, B. M. and Williams, C. B. (1978) Colonoscopy for unexplained rectal bleeding. *Br. Med. J.*, **2**, 1685–7.

22. Williams, C. B. (1973) Diathermy – biopsy: a technique of endoscopic management of small polyps. *Endoscopy*, **5**, 215–18.

23. Hunt, R. H. and Buchanan, J. D. (1981) The diagnosis and management of mucosal angiodysplasia. *Gastrointest. Endosc.*, **27**, 123.

24. Bourdette, D. and Greenberg, B. (1979) Twelve-year history of gastrointestinal bleeding in a patient with calcific aortic stenosis and haemorrhagic telangiectasia. *Dig. Dis. Sci.*, **24**, 77–82.

25. Roberts, L. K., Gold, R. E. and Routt, W. E. (1981) Gastric angiodysplasia. *Radiology*, **139**, 355–9.

26. Weaver, G. A., Alpern, H. D., Davis, J. S., Ramsay, W. H. and Reichelderfer, M. (1979) Gastrointestinal angiodysplasia associated with aortic valve disease: part of a spectrum of angiodysplasia of the gut. *Gastroenterology*, **77**, 1–11.

27. Miller, K. D., Tutton, R. H., Bell, K. A. and Simon, B. K. (1979) Angiodysplasia of the colon. *Radiology*, **132**, 309–13.

28. Baum, S., Athanasoulis, C. A. and Waltman, A. (1972) Acquired vascular ectasias of caecum and right colon as a cause of chronic gastrointestinal bleeding. *58th Sci. Meet. Radiol. Soc. N. Am.*, *(Chicago)*, **Essay 181**.

29. Wangensteen, O. H. (1955) *Intestinal Obstruction*, 3rd edn, C. C. Thomas Publications, Springfield, Illinois.

30. Galloway, S. J., Casarella, W. J. and Shimkin, P. M. (1974) Vascular malformations of the right colon as a cause of bleeding in patients with aortic stenosis. *Radiology*, **113**, 11–15.

31. Mitsudo, S. M., Boley, S. J., Brandt, L. J., Montefusco, C. M. and Sammartano, R. J. (1979) Vascular ectasias of the right colon in the elderly: a district pathological entity. *Human Pathol.*, **10**, 5, 585–600.

32. Giacchino, J. L., Geis, W. P., Pickleman, J. R., Dado, D. V. *et al.* (1979) Changing perspectives in massive lower intestinal haemorrhage. *Surgery*, **86**, 368–76.

33. Howard, O. M., Buchanan, J. D. and Hunt, R. H. (1982) Angiodysplasia of the colon: Experience of 26 cases. *Lancet*, **ii**, 16–18.

34. Hunt, R. H. and Teague, R. H. (1980) Vascular abnormalities of the colon. *Proc. Third Asian Pac. Congr. Dig. Endosc.*, Taiwan, 132–5.

35. Moore, J. D., Thompson, N. W., Appelman, H. D. and Foley, D. (1976) Arteriovenous malformations of the gastrointestinal tract. *Arch. Surg.*, **3**, 381–9.

36. Sing, A. K., Agenant, D. M. A., Hausman, R. and Tijtgat, G. N. (1980) Vascular ectasias (angiodysplasias) of the caecum and the ascending colon. *Fortschrip. Roetgenstr.*, **1321**, 534–41.

37. Heyde, E. C. (1958) Gastrointestinal bleeding in aortic stenosis. *New Eng. J. Med.*, **259**, 196–200.

38. Williams, R. C., Jr. (1961) Aortic stenosis and unexplained gastrointestinal bleeding. *Arch. Intern. Med.*, **108**, 859–63.

39. Boss, E. G. and Rosenbaum, J. M. (1971) Bleeding from the right colon associated with aortic stenosis. *Am. J. Dig. Dis.*, **16**, 269–75.

40. Cass, A. J., Bliss, B. P., Bolton, R. P. and Cooper, B. T. (1980) Gastrointestinal bleeding, angiodysplasia of the colon and acquired Von Willebrand's disease. *Br. J. Surg.*, **67**, 639–41.

41. Ramsay, D. M., MacLeod, D. A. D., Buist, T. A. S. and Heading, R. C. (1976) Persistent gastrointestinal bleeding due to angiodysplasia of the gut in Von Willebrand's disease. *Lancet*, **ii**, 275–8.

42. Rosborough, T. K. and Swain, W. R. (1978) Acquired Von Willebrand's disease, platelet release defect and angiodysplasia. *Am. J. Med.*, **65**, 96–100.

43. Baum, S., Athanasoulis, C. A., Waltman, A. C., Galdabini, J. J. *et al.* (1977) Angiodysplasia of the right colon: a cause of gastrointestinal bleeding. *Am. J. Roentgenol.*, **129**, 789–94.

44. Talman, E. A., Dixon, D. S. and Gutierrez, F. E. (1979) Role of arteriography in rectal haemorrhage due to arteriovenous malformations and diverticulosis. *Ann. Surg.*, **190**, 203–13.

45. Tarin, D., Allison, D. J., Modlin, I. M. and Neale, G. (1978) Diagnosis and management of obscure gastrointestinal bleeding. *Br. Med. J.*, **2**, 751–4.

46. Boley, S. J., Sprayregan, S., Sammartano, R. J., Adamas, A. and Kleinhause, S. (1977) The pathophysiologic basis for the angiographic signs of vascular ectasias of the colon. *Diagn. Radiol.*, **125**, 615–21.

47. Heald, R. J. and Ray, J. E. (1974) Vascular malformations of the intestine: an important cause of obscure gastrointestinal haemorrhage. *South. Med. J.*, **67**, 33–8.
48. Bowden, T. A., Hooks, V. H. and Mansberger, A. R. (1979) Intraoperative gastrointestinal endoscopy. *Ann. Surg.*, **191**, 680–7.
49. Forde, K. A. (1981) Intraoperative Colonoscopy in *Colonoscopy, Techniques, Clinical Practice and Colour Atlas*, (eds R. H. Hunt and J. D. Waye), Chapman and Hall, London, pp. 189–98.
50. Buchanan, J. D. and Hunt, R. H. (1980) Photography and coagulation biopsy confirm the diagnosis of angiodysplasia. *Gut*, **21**, 10.
51. Nagy, G. S. (1981) in *Colonoscopy, Techniques, Clinical Practice and Colour Atlas*, (eds R. H. Hunt and J. D. Waye), Chapman and Hall, London, pp. 19–26.
52. Taylor, E. W., Bentley, S., Youngs, D. and Keighley, M. R. B. (1981) Bowel preparation and the safety of colonoscopic polypectomy. *Gastroenterology*, **81**, 1–4.
53. Menanteau, B., Amselle, M., Bonnet, F., Ducreux, A. and Senecail, B. (1980) Angiodysplasic du colon droit. *J. Radiol.*, **61**, 717–21.
54. Allison, D. J. and Hemingway, A. P. (1981) Angiodysplasia: does old age begin at nineteen? *Lancet*, **ii**, 979–80.
55. Tadavarthy, S. M., Castaneda-Zuniga, W., Zollikofer, C., Nemer, F. *et al.* (1981) Angiodysplasia of the right colon treated by embolisation with Ivalon (polyvinyl alcohol). *Cardiovasc. Intervent. Radiol.*, **4**, 39–42.
56. Richardson, J. D., Max, M. H. and Fling, L. M. (1978) Bleeding vascular malformations of the intestine. *Surgery*, **84**, 430–6.

Section B

OESOPHAGEAL PROBLEMS

II

Dysphagia – an overview

G. N. J. TYTGAT and J. F. W. M. BARTELSMAN

Dysphagia is defined as difficulty in swallowing a liquid or solid bolus with hindering in the passage at any point between the oral cavity and the stomach. Dysphagia occurs only during the act of swallowing. This means that the sensation of altered or delayed passage of fluid or food will be felt within some 10 seconds after the onset of a swallow.

When an abnormality develops in the complex act of swallowing, the patient becomes aware of this process and seeks medical help. The patient may feel to be unable to initiate a swallow because his tongue fails to push the bolus into the hypopharynx or fluid may regurgitate through his nose and lead to aspiration. In others, dysphagia is characterized by a sensation of retrosternal fullness or pressure, transient sticking of food during its passage, or the sensation of a complete hold of food or fluid.

Dysphagia may be associated with painful sensations but should be differentiated from odynophagia, which is pain upon swallowing without delay in the transit of food.

Dysphagia is perhaps one of the most specific and reliable symptoms in gastrointestinal disease. Every effort should therefore be made to determine its cause. By thorough evaluation of the history and the use of several simple diagnostic methods, the aetiology can almost always be established.

PHYSIOLOGY OF SWALLOWING

The oropharyngeal stage of swallowing requires complex co-ordination of neuromuscular functions of the oropharynx. During this stage, which lasts approximately one second, the tongue moves up and back, the tonsillar pillars contract, the soft palate rises, the larynx moves anteriorly and the cricopharyngeal muscle relaxes as the posterior pharyngeal constrictor muscle contracts to push the bolus downward into the oesophagus. The second stage begins as the bolus enters the cervical oesophagus, upon which a primary oesophageal peristaltic contraction wave begins. This primary peristalsis pushes the bolus by sequential contractions towards the distal oesophagus at a rate of $3-4$ cm s^{-1}. As the peristaltic wave approaches the distal oesophagus, the lower oesophageal sphincter has already begun to relax, facilitating its emptying into the stomach. Oesophageal emptying is usually completed within about eight seconds of the onset of swallowing.

PATHOPHYSIOLOGY AND AETIOLOGICAL CONSIDERATIONS

Patients with dysphagia fall into two main categories: pre-oesophageal or oropharyngeal dysphagia and oesophageal dysphagia. It is convenient in differential considerations to categorize dysphagia into two broad classes: (a) that due to primary neuromuscular disturbances, such as failure of peristalsis or inco-ordination of peristalsis and sphincter function and (b) that due to mechanical obstruction in and around the oesophagus. In general terms, about 50% or more of the effective luminal diameter must be lost before dysphagia will appear in many patients.

Pre-oesophageal dysphagia is almost always the result of neuromuscular disease such as pseudobulbar paresis due to cerebrovascular disease, cricopharyngeal dysfunction, myotonic dystrophy, myasthenia gravis, amyotrophic lateral sclerosis, dermatomyositis, muscular dystrophy, bulbar poliomyelitis, Parkinson's disease etc. Vascular lesions involving the brain stem are undoubtedly the most common cause of dysphagia amongst these entities. Less common causes of pre-oesophageal dysphagia are tumours, such as cancers of the piriform sinus or thyroid enlargement or malignancy, or inflammatory lesions of the pharynx and tonsils. A not unusual cause of pre-oesophageal dysphagia is the presence of a pharyngo-oesophageal or Zenker's diverticulum which may be associated with cricopharyngeal inco-ordination.

Also at the level of the oesophagus proper we distinguish primary neuromuscular disturbances and mechanical obstruction. In the primary neuromuscular disturbances, the most common diseases are achalasia, scleroderma, and related collagen vascular diseases, diffuse oesophageal spasm and related disorders, and a miscellaneous group including diabetes mellitus, alcoholism, Chagas' disease and presbyoesophagus.

In the list of mechanical obstructions in or around the oesophagus one may differentiate between intrinsic and extrinsic oesophageal causes. Most common intrinsic causes for mechanical obstruction are malignant or benign tumours, inflammatory strictures due to reflux, ingestion of corrosive agents or sutureline strictures, severe oesophageal inflammation such as due to herpes, candida or pill-oesophagitis, lower oesophageal rings such as Schatzki rings and oesophageal webbs, diverticular formation, duplication cysts etc.

Extrinsic causes for oesophageal obstruction are vascular compression such as dysphagia lusoria, extensive tortuosity and elongation of the thoracic vessels, mediastinal tumours or nodes, peri-oesophageal mediastinal fibrosis such as secondary to blunt chest trauma or postsurgery, such as postvagotomy or postfundoplication, foreign bodies and pronounced cervical osteoarthritis [1, 2].

COMMON SYNDROMES OF DYSPHAGIA

The benign stricture syndrome

Stricture formation may be expected in 10–15% of patients with reflux oesophagitis. Recurring circumferential mucosal erosion and ulceration finally produces scarring and retraction. Such strictures are usually located in the distal third just proximal to the gastro-oesophageal junction except in cases of an endobrachyoesophagus where a highly located stricture may be seen in over half the patients. Peptic strictures usually have a smooth tapered appearance and are of variable length. They rarely if ever close the lumen completely. Peptic strictures usually produce no symptoms until the luminal diameter is reduced to about 12–13 mm or less. Then the patient begins to note the symptoms of dysphagia when ingesting solid food but not liquids. Characteristically there is associated pain or discomfort on impact of the bolus. Initially the block is often intermittent. Such dysphagia should be distinguished from cervical dysphagia or a sensation of a lump in the throat which may be the initial complaint in reflux oesophagitis.

It is not uncommon for the patient to notice improvement of his usual reflux symptoms of heartburn and regurgitation as he develops dysphagia. If the stricture is sufficiently narrow to produce persistent dysphagia, heartburn is rarely present (Fig. 11.1). In addition there usually is no pain between meals. Often, however, the oesophagus remains sensitive to hot drinks or alcohol.

If the process progresses unchecked, even ingestion of liquids may become problematic but progression is usually slow.

The neoplastic narrowing

The dysphagia of oesophageal cancer is usually of gradual onset and of steadily increasing severity. Malignant dysphagia usually develops when about half the circumference of the oesophagus is invaded and appears to be associated initially with inco-ordination of oesophageal contraction. About 50% or more of the effective oesophageal luminal diameter must be lost before dysphagia will finally appear in the majority of patients. This fact explains why oesophageal cancer is usually well advanced when first diagnosed in many patients.

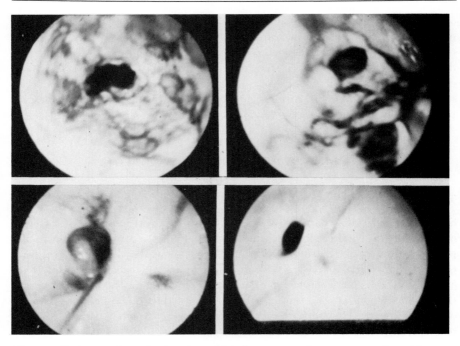

Fig. 11.1 Early oesophageal stricturing with inflammatory changes contrasting with a non-inflamed narrow stricture below as seen in longstanding gastro-oesophageal reflux disease.

At first the patient notices difficulty in swallowing such foodstuffs as meat and apple. This gradually increases until finally it may be impossible for the patient to swallow his own saliva. Since the rate of flow of a liquid through a tube is proportional to the fourth power of its radius, a small further encroachment by a growth causes a large increase in dysphagia when the effective luminal diameter is reduced to a few millimetres. In other patients there may be a sudden total obstruction owing to impaction of a bolus of food.

Pain is not a prominent feature, except in the later stages when local spread has occurred. When pain is present, it is usually related to the lower end of the sternum and may radiate through the back.

There usually is no sensitivity to hot drinks or alcohol.

The neuromuscular dysfunction syndrome

The diagnosis of a motor abnormality such as achalasia and/or diffuse oesophageal spasm is usually indicated by the insidious onset of symptoms although at times onset can be dramatically sudden. Characteristically there is equal difficulty for solid foods and liquids. Usually progression is slow over months.

Dysphagia is often associated with regurgitation of indigested food, hours to days after ingestion together with a sensation of middle or lower substernal fullness. The tasteless sometimes quite voluminous regurgitated fluid corresponds to recently drunk fluid or thick saliva which tend to float on the other contents in the oesophagus.

Typical impact pain is usually absent. On the other hand spontaneous chest pain unrelated to meals may be present.

SCORING SYSTEM

Increasingly a scoring system for swallowing capabilities as summarized in Table 11.1 is used. Grade 1 is diagnosed when the patient is unable to swallow certain solid foods, such as meat and apple; grade 2 is diagnosed when only semi-solid soft or only blenderized food can be swallowed; in grade 3 only liquids can be consumed; grade 4 is diagnosed when the patient is unable to swallow even liquids in adequate amounts, necessitating parenteral administration of fluids to prevent dehydration [3, 4].

Table 11.1 Dysphagia — scoring systems

From Atkinson *et al.* [3]	From Stoller *et al.* [4]
0: taking normal diet	0: any foods
1: unable to swallow certain solids	1: all soft foods
2: limited to semi-solid soft diet	2: blenderized foods
3: liquids only	3: clear liquids only
4: unable to swallow even liquids in adequate amounts – intravenous fluid needed	4: nothing (not even saliva)

HISTORY TAKING IN PATIENTS WITH DYSPHAGIA

History is a most valuable tool in the evaluation of a patient with dysphagia and should lead to a strong suspicion of the correct diagnosis in perhaps over 90% of patients. As shown below there are several pertinent questions to be asked [5, 6].

1. Where do you feel the bolus sticks?

Patients with pre-oesophageal dysphagia complain of food sticking in the throat. Patients with oesophageal dysphagia note food sticking somewhere between the xyphoid and the suprasternal notch. If the patient localizes his sticking sensation along the sternum, often, but not always, a reasonable or good correlation with the obstructing site may be found. Conversely if the symptom is localized to the suprasternal notch, there is often poor correlation with the anatomic site. Indeed lesions in the lower oesophagus such as early malignancy or gastro-oesophageal reflux disease, may occasionally cause a sensation of upper suprasternal dysphagia. According to Edwards [7] the patient is wrong more often than he is right in localizing the precise site of the problem because stimulation of receptors tend to be referred to individually variable places. This author feels that patients are more accurate in estimating the time interval between the swallow and the sensation of impact. Mechanical obstruction at the level of the body of the oesophagus usually causes dysphagia within 2–5 seconds whereas distal obstruction may be perceived after 8–10 seconds.

2. Is there equal difficulty with liquids and solids?
When dysphagia is greater for solids than for liquids, a structural disorder, intrinsic or extrinsic to the oesophagus, is usually found. Equal difficulty early in the course of dysphagia usually indicates a motor disorder rather than luminal narrowing.

3. Is concomitant regurgitation present?
When associated with pre-oesophageal swallowing difficulty, sometimes with bulging and gurgling of the neck with drinks, regurgitation of undigested food hours to days after ingestion suggests a pharyngo-oesophageal Zenker's diverticulum. When this type of regurgitation occurs with middle or lower substernal fullness, achalasia is likely.

4. How long has the dysphagia been present?
Chronic dysphagia of many years duration is most consistent with a motor disorder such as achalasia. Cancer usually presents as a constant and inexorably progressive dysphagia that usually evolves quite rapidly. Benign strictures may present rather similarly though a longer course of development is more characteristic.

5. How often does dysphagia occur?
Dysphagia secondary to an inflammatory fibrous process may sometimes behave variably from meal to meal, in contrast with the constancy of dysphagia in case of malignant narrowing. Truly intermittent, acute or recurrent, dysphagia, often occurring over many years, sometimes with long symptom-free intervals between episodes, usually implies the existence of a ring or web. A web generally occurs high in the oesophagus with symptoms referred to the neck. A Schatzki ring usually causes dysphagia when its diameter is narrowed to 13 mm or less but occasionally even with a larger diameter between 13 and 20 mm intermittent dysphagia may occur. Symptoms attributable to mucosal rings usually occur during ingestion of a partially masticated solid bolus, often steak, usually eaten in a social setting (steakhouse syndrome).

6. Is there pain upon swallowing?

Pain upon swallowing may be associated with motor disorders. When an ingested bolus sticks in the middle or lower oesophagus and causes pain that is relieved by regurgitation or by passing of the bolus, the diagnosis of diffuse spasm is likely. The pain of achalasia and diffuse spasm may also occur in the absence of dysphagia. Pain upon swallowing may also occur in the presence of severe oesophagitis such as infection with herpes or candida, in the presence of oesophageal ulceration, in tumours with mediastinal invasion, and in instances of peri-oesophageal inflammation. Drug-induced oesophagitis or pill oesophagitis is an increasingly recognized cause of rather acute painful dysphagia. Potassium chloride, tetracycline, quinidine, ferrous sulphate and emepronium bromide are most commonly incriminated drugs,. The corrosive nature of these drugs added to delay in clearing from the oesophagus, especially in prone position [8], may initiate chemically-induced oesophageal mucosal damage (Fig. 11.2).

7. Is foodsticking painful?

Obstruction by a food bolus at the level of a stricture causes a sensation of pressure or impact pain which is more pronounced for an inflamed fibrous stricture than for a neoplastic one.

8. Is spontaneous chest pain present?

In motor disorders there often is chest pain, unrelated to swallowing food.

9. Is coughing or wheezing present?

Coughing or wheezing may suggest oesophageal stasis and nocturnal aspiration or severe gastro-oesophageal reflux. Such a subtle but potentially severe problem of

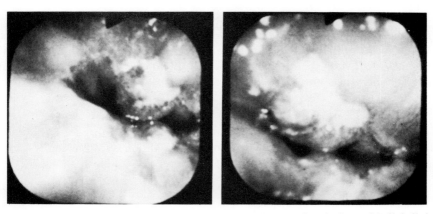

Fig. 11.2 Example of 'pill-oesophagitis' with focal necrosis of the epithelial lining surrounded by marked inflammatory changes.

aspiration with coughing spells, chronic laryngobronchitis or nocturnal asthma may be the major or only complaint volunteered by the patient.

Tracheo-oesophageal fistula from oesophageal or bronchogenic cancer may also present with cough and aspiration pneumonia.

When aspiration is chronic, pulmonary fibrosis and symptoms of respiratory insufficiency may result.

10. Has there been weight loss?

Any of the diseases associated with progressive or recurrent forms of dysphagia may result in weight loss. Profound weight loss within a short period is however more suggestive of cancer than of any other disease.

11. Does the food stick while the patient is eating or does this sensation occur only after the end of the meal?

Food sticking during the meal is usually indicative of organic obstruction whereas food sticking after the meal is to be considered as a referred sensation of paraesthesia.

12. Did reflux symptoms, such as heartburn, precede dysphagia or has heartburn been otherwise associated with this dysphagia?

Heartburn preceding the development of dysphagia and abating at its onset usually indicates a benign oesophageal stricture. Also achalasia may occasionally be accompanied by a burning retrosternal sensation.

13. Does hot drink or alcohol burn upon swallowing?

A burning sensation is indicative of sensitivity of the oesophageal lining as usually seen in reflux oesophagitis.

14. Is skin disease associated with dysphagia?

The distal two-thirds of the oesophagus are involved in up to 80% of patients with scleroderma. Tylosis (keratosis palmaris et plantaris) is associated with an increased incidence of oesophageal cancer.

15. Is oral disease present?

Xerostomia is a major clinical manifestation of Sjögren's syndrome. The latter is often associated with other collagen disorders. In addition xerostomia may lead to insufficient lubrication of the swallowed bolus.

16. Does the history indicate cardiac disease?

A huge left atrium may occasionally compress the oesophagus to such extent that it produces dysphagia. Similarly large aneurysms of the aortic arch or descending aorta may dislocate or compress the oesophagus.

17. Is neuromuscular disease present?
Dermatomyositis with characteristic muscle weakness and dermatological manifestations may also affect the musculature of the proximal third of the oesophagus,
causing dysphagia and not infrequently aspiration. In addition, the cricopharyngeal sphincter may be atonic.

Cricopharyngeal inco-ordination, such as incomplete relaxation or premature
contraction before the end of the pharyngeal contraction wave (Fig. 11.3) may be
associated with a Zenker's diverticulum, Parkinsonism, amyotrophic lateral
sclerosis, pseudobulbar palsy or myasthenia gravis.

18. Does the history indicate previous abdominal surgery?
Any manipulation of the gastro-oesophageal junction may predispose to dysphagia. Postsurgical dysphagia may occur when a fundoplication is too tight or has
slipped creating a telescope phenomenon. Fibrosis around the cardia is another
major cause of dysphagia usually for solids. After nasogastric intubation a fibrotic
stenosis may occur when the aspiration of the stomach is inadequate especially in a
supine hypersecretive patient.

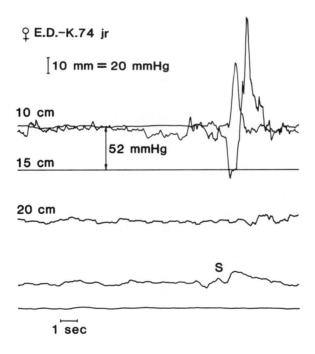

Fig. 11.3 Example of dyskinesia of the upper oesophageal sphincter, characterized by
premature closure of the cricopharyngeal muscle before the end of the pharyngeal
contraction wave.

19. Does the history indicate ingestion of lye?
Lye or corrosive ingestion may precede the development of a fibrous stricture by a long time. Moreover a lye burn may predispose to oesophageal malignancy.

20. Is osteoarthritis present?
Cervical spurs from severe osteoarthritis may, though rarely, impinge on the upper oesophagus and produce intermittent dysphagia, sometimes related to neck position (Fig. 11.4).

ROLE OF ENDOSCOPY IN THE DIFFERENTIAL DIAGNOSIS OF DYSPHAGIA

Endoscopy is most useful in differentiating carcinoma from other constricting lesions such as benign tumours or inflammatory lesions.

The macroscopic appearance of advanced oesophageal cancer is well known. Although many combined or transitional forms exist, in general three main gross types may be distinguished.

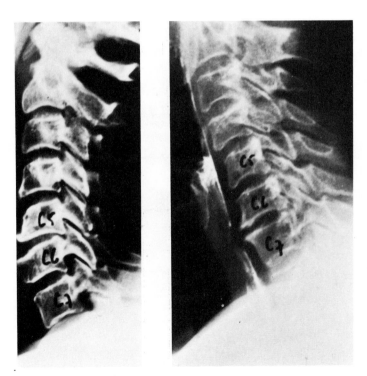

Fig. 11.4 Examples of pronounced osteoarthritic changes around C6.

(a) The exophytic polypous growth is often bulky, cauliflower like, wide-based and usually reveals a coarsely nodular, haemorrhagic surface with or without additional erosive or ulcerative defects.

(b) The ulcerative type is mainly characterized by a central meniscoid-type necrosis, surrounded by heaping edges; usually a major part of the circumference is involved, leading often to early circular tumourous narrowing.

(c) Diffusely infiltrating scirrhous cancers manifest obvious thickening and rigidity of a variable length of the oesophageal wall, with fixation of the irregularly thickened, coarsely nodular, rarely ulcerated mucosa to the deeper layers.

Very important for the differential diagnosis are multiple-aimed biopsies. No problems are to be expected for histological diagnosis of polypoid tumours or for meniscoid lesions where the proximal tumour edge is clearly visible. Preferably a Ch-7 biopsy forceps with a central spike should be used for tangential lesions. Not only the malignancy but any proximal mural irregularity should be biopsied in order to detect intramural metastases (Fig. 11.5).

Still problematic, however, are stenotic lesions. It is often difficult if not impossible to make an exact endoscopic diagnosis. Only multiple biopsies or cytology may clarify the true nature of the lesion but even that may be problematic. Moderately severe narrowings should be studied with a small calibre endoscope. Usually the lesion can be passed so that biopsies can be obtained not only from the proximal edge but also from within the lesion. Very tight stenoses cannot be passed with any type of endoscope. Only guided biopsies can be obtained from the upper edge. Small nodular elevations with whitish yellowish discoloration or tiny erosive changes or areas around fistulous openings should be biopsied preferentially. Because of the submucosal extension of the tumour, biopsies may often only show secondary inflammatory changes. The diagnostic yield can occasionally be improved by introducing the biopsy forceps blindly into the strictured area in order to sample the deeper sites but unfortunately this is not always successful. In such circumstances it may be important to obtain cytological material using a nylon cytology brush which may usually be passed inside the lesion. An alternative method is to gently dilate the stricture up to 10–12 mm in order to allow taking guided biopsies from inside and also from below the lesion using a small calibre endoscope.

Achalasia-mimicking submucosal malignancies such as illustrated in Fig. 11.6, are very problematic. Such lesions can usually be passed with a small calibre endoscope. Not infrequently, no endoscopic abnormalities are visible and tiny superficial biopsies reveal only normal squamous or gastric mucosa. One way to solve such problems is to use large biopsy forceps, sampling tissue from the same site until the deeper layers of the submucosa are obtained [9].

In the majority of the studies a correct histological diagnosis is possible, often in over 90% of patients provided more than 6 biopsies are taken (Table 11.2). The higher the number of biopsies the higher the chances of hitting non-necrotic tumour tissue. It is not uncommon that more than 12 biopsies are needed but even then occasionally no correct tissue diagnosis can be obtained (Fig. 11.7). Cytology also reaches a high diagnostic accuracy. Both techniques are therefore complementary. The better the biopsy results, the lesser the need for additional cytology. A disadvantage of cytology is the presence of a small percentage of false positives in virtually all published series [23].

PITFALLS IN DIFFERENTIAL DIAGNOSIS

Any physician responsible for diagnosis and care of patients with dysphagia must develop a complete up-to-date differential diagnosis, if he is to minimize diagnostic errors.

An incomplete history may be thoroughly misleading. In addition attention

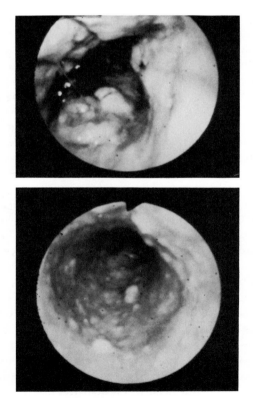

Fig. 11.5 Tiny whitish mucosal nodules due to intramural metastasis from a more distally located malignancy.

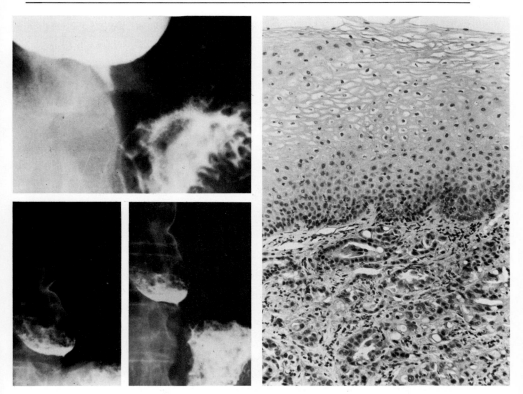

Fig. 11.6 Distal submucosal malignancy mimicking achalasia. The lesion could easily be passed with a small calibre endoscope. Multiple (tiny) biopsies without abnormality were taken before referral for pneumodilatation. Deep submucosal biopsies with a large biopsy forceps revealed the submucosal malignancy.

should be given to rarities such as hiccups as a predominant symptom of oesophageal obstruction instead of dysphagia [24].

One should be extremely reluctant in accepting that dysphagia is of psychogenic origin. The physician must be ever mindful that this symptom does not occur on an emotional basis and therefore must make every effort to determine its cause.

One should not accept a negative barium swallow as final examination in a patient with dysphagia.

A common error is to challenge the oesophagus only in upright position with liquid barium and not with a solid bolus or in the supine position (Fig. 11.8).

Failure to perform a complete examination may be disastrous. An examination limited to the pharynx and upper oesophagus in patients with mid or distal lesions, who refer the symptoms of dysphagia to the suprasternal notch, the neck or the back of the throat, will lead to a mistaken diagnosis.

Table 11.2 Diagnostic accuracy of biopsy and cytology of oesophagocardiac malignancy

	No. Ca patients	No. biopsies	% positive biopsies	% positive cytology	% positive biopsies and cytology
Nakamura et al., 1968 [10]			85		
Kobayashi et al., 1970 [11, 12]	8	>3	88	100	
Prolla, 1973 [13]	25	3–4	72	92	
Seifert and Atay, 1975 [14]	64		81		
Winawer et al., 1975 [15]	30	4	66	97	
Bruni and Nelson, 1975 [16]	103	6–8	94	87	
Hishon et al., 1976 [17]	20		50	90	
Witzel et al., 1976 [18]	47	6–10	77	89	
Prolla et al., 1977 [19]	73	6–8	78	89	
Gütz and Wildner, 1978 [20]	75	—	93		
Eastman et al., 1978 [21]	69	—	71	76	
Mortensen et al., 1981 [22]	36	—	81	86	92
Amsterdam series	300	8–12	97		

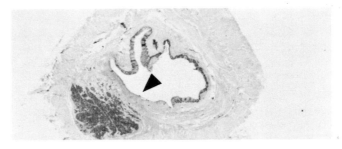

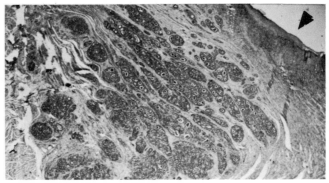

Fig. 11.7 Illustration of the limitations of biopsy and cytology. Endoscopically there was only a tiny erosion in the distal oesophagus. As can be seen, cancerous tissue is present only in the deeper layers not sampled with the standard small size biopsy forceps.

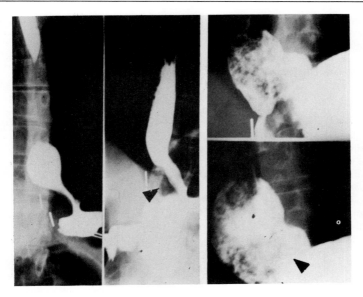

Fig. 11.8 Example of a patient with postfundoplication dysphagia. No abnormalities were apparently detected when studied with liquid barium in the upright position. However, when challenged with a meat bolus, striking dilatation and slow emptying of the oesophagus was easily detectable.

Failure to use manometry or scintigraphy and failure to use adequate endoscopy are not unusual causes of diagnostic error.

Foreign bodies should always be ruled out, especially in children and in the elderly. Older people do not always complain or dysphagia but instead just stop eating. Luminal patency should always be checked first before extensive work-ups for anorexia and weightloss are decided upon.

REFERENCES

1. Castell, D. O., Knuff, T. E., Brown, F. C., Gerhardt, D. C., Burns, T. W. and Gaskins, R. D. (1979) Dysphagia. *Gastroenterology*, **76**, 1015–24.
2. Phillips, M. M. and Hendrix, T. R. (1971) Dysphagia. *Postgrad. Med. J.*, **47**, 81–6.
3. Atkinson, M., Ferguson, R. and Ogilvie, A. C. (1979) Management of malignant dysphagia by intubation at endoscopy. *J. R. Soc. Med.*, **27**, 894–7.
4. Stoller, J. L., Samer, K. J., Toppin, D. I. and Flores, A. D. (1977) Carcinoma of the esophagus: A new proposal for the evaluation of treatment. *Can. J. Surg.*, **20**, 454–9.
5. Boyce, H. W., Jr. (1982) Personal communication.
6. Gambescia, R. A. and Rogers, A. I. (1976) Dysphagia – diagnosis by history. *Postgrad. Med.*, **59**, 211–16.
7. Edwards, D. A. W. (1976) Discriminatory value of symptoms in the differential diagnosis of dysphagia. *Clin. Gastroenterol.*, **5**, 49–57.

8. Evans, K. T. and Roberts, G. M. (1976) Where do all the tablets go? *Lancet*, **ii**, 1237–9.
9. Tucker, H. J., Snape, W. J. Jr. and Cohen, S. (1978) Achalasia secondary to carcinoma, manometric and clinical features. *Ann. Int. Med.*, **89**, 315–18.
10. Nakamura, Y., Arimori, M. and Kumagai, Y. (1968) Examination with esophagoscopes: utilization of the fiberscope. *Stomach Intestine*, **3**, 1361–8.
11. Kobayashi, S., Prolla, J. C. and Kirsner, J. B. (1970) Brushing cytology of the esophagus and stomach under direct vision by fiberscopes. *Acta Cytol.*, **14**, 219–23.
12. Kobayashi, S., Prolla, J. C., Winans, C. S. and Kirsner, J. B. (1970) Improved endoscopic diagnosis of gastroesophageal malignancy. Combined use of direct vision brushing cytology and biopsy. *J. Am. Med. Assoc.*, **212**, 2086–9.
13. Prolla, J. C. (1973) Cancer of the gastrointestinal tract. I. Esophagus. Histopathology and cytology in detection. *J. Am. Med. Assoc.*, **226**, 1554–6.
14. Seifert, E. and Atay, Z. (1975) *Maligne Tumoren des Gastrointestinaltraktes. Fortschritte der Endoskopie*. Thieme, Stuttgart.
15. Winawer, S. J., Sherlock, P. and Belladonna, J. (1975) Endoscopic brush cytology in oesophageal cancer. *J. Am. Med. Assoc.*, **232**, 1358–60.
16. Bruni, H. C. and Nelson, R. S. (1975) Carcinoma of the esophagus and cardia. Diagnostic evaluation in 113 cases. *J. Thorac. Cardiovasc. Surg.*, **70**, 367–70.
17. Hishon, S., Lovell, D. and Gummer, J. W. P. (1976) Cytology in the diagnosis of oesophageal cancer. *Lancet*, **i**, 296–7.
18. Witzel, L., Halter, F., Grétillat, P. A., Scheuer, U. and Keller, M. (1976) Evaluation of specific value of endoscopic biopsies and brush cytology for malignancies of the oesophagus and stomach. *Gut*, **17**, 375–7.
19. Prolla, J. C., Reilley, R. W. and Kirsner, J. B. (1977) Direct vision endoscopic cytology and biopsy in the diagnosis of esophageal and gastric tumours: current experience. *Acta Cytol.*, **21**, 399–402.
20. Gütz, H. J. and Wildner, G. P. (1978) Die diagnostiche Sicherheit von Endoscopie und Biopsie bei stenosierenden Prozessen in Ösophagus und Kardia. *Dtsch. Z. Verdau. Stoffwechselkr.*, **38**, 47–9.
21. Eastman, M. C., Gear, M. W. L. and Nicol, A. (1978) An assessment of the accuracy of modern endoscopic diagnosis of oesophageal stricture. *Br. J. Surg.*, **65**, 182–5.
22. Mortensen, N. J. and Mackenzie, E. F. D. (1981) Accuracy of oesophageal brush cytology: results of a prospective study and multicentre slide exchange. *Br. J. Surg.*, **68**, 513–15.
23. Hughes, H. E., Lee, F. D. and Mackenzie, T. F. (1978) Endoscopic cytology and biopsy in the upper gastro-intestinal tract. *Clin. Gastroenterol.*, **7**, 375–96.
24. Kaufmann, H. J. (1982) Hiccups: An occasional sign of esophageal obstruction. *Gastroenterology*, **82**, 1443–5.

12

Motility disorders of the oesophagus

D. A. W. EDWARDS

In the context of this chapter 'motility disorders' includes: (a) disturbances of muscle contraction and relaxation and of the motor supply to the oesophagus and (b) a decrease in compliance, that is, an increase in the resistance to stretch of the wall of the oesophagus and surrounding structures, e.g. in benign strictures, and abnormalities in elastance, that is, the forces tending to return the wall to its original length after it has been stretched, e.g. the achalasic sphincter and post-hiatal repair dysphagia.

SYMPTOMS

Many motility disorders of the oesophagus seen by the radiologist are not associated with symptoms, for example, 'tertiary contractions' and the dilated or weakly contracting oesophagus of old age, or motor neurone disease. The loss of peristalsis associated with smooth muscle destruction in systemic sclerosis does not cause symptoms but can be an important clue to the presence of that systemic disease. In achalasia also it is not the loss of the peristaltic wave which causes the dysphagia, but the obstruction resulting from the reduction in relaxation of the sphincter. Most patients present for investigation with symptoms, however, rather than an abnormal barium swallow.

Chest pain unassociated with any dysphagia is a common diagnostic problem, some of it still unsolved. Obstructive dysphagia is the more common symptom, and needs to be subdivided into (a) true obstruction where there is radiographic demonstration of obstruction to food or drink, and (b) false obstruction where the lumen is seen to open to a normal width when challenged with liquid barium. False obstruction is further subdivided into (i) pseudodysphagia, a paraesthesiae;

and (ii) 'tender oesophagus'. The paraesthesia is a sensation that food is sticking, or sitting somewhere in the midline between the thyroid cartilage and the epigastrium, which is not present when the patient is eating or drinking, but develops 10–110 minutes after and lasts from minutes to hours. There is no specific abnormality visible endoscopically or radiologically. 'Tender oesophagus' is the state of part of the oesophageal wall which is unusually sensitive to stretch. The sensation produced by a bolus passing through persists for minutes to hours after the stimulus has gone. Because of the sensation, which is worse the faster the patient drinks, and the larger or more solid the bolus, the patient feels that they are packing more and more into the oesophagus and that the bolus is not passing into the stomach. They may feel the oesophagus is so full that they deliberately regurgitate. Endoscopically and radiologically the oesophagus is normal.

True obstructive dysphagia is sometimes misunderstood by radiologists and endoscopists. The patient is right more often than the physician, who may not get all the details of the history. The physician is likely to be right more often than the radiologist who may miss causes of obstruction if he does not stretch the normal wall to its full extent and thereby show the increased resistance to stretch of the abnormal area. The radiologist is likely to be right more often than the endoscopist who may easily fail to *observe* and interpret a cause for obstruction of food or drink, and may easily fail to *feel* one. To the patient an achalasic sphincter, extrinsic compression, submucosal neoplastic infiltration, post-vagotomy peri-oesophagitis and post-hiatal repair constriction are all causes of obstruction of liquid, let alone solid, yet an endoscope may pass through easily. The patient finds that a peptic stricture obstructs food, yet, except for old and dense ones, the majority of peptic strictures are missed by the majority of endoscopists because they cannot *feel* them. The patient's definition of an obstruction is something which holds up food or drink; the surgeon's and endoscopist's definition is something which holds up the endoscope or bougie. Proper radiology will demonstrate what the patient feels if a true obstruction is present (see below).

Benign strictures and early malignant strictures do not slow down the rate of drinking because the lumen is open to several millimetres. The wall resists stretch enough to obstruct the flow of food, particles above a certain size, or a bolus of small particles which glue together e.g. dry flaked fish, overcooked rice, and stiff mashed potatoes. The patient therefore has dysphagia for solids but not liquids. The lumen in achalasia is closed to liquid as well as solid, but is a muscular closure which can be stretched by building up intra-oesophageal pressure to open to 1–4 mm. This sometimes allows liquid to be drunk at a normal speed, e.g. a standard challenge of 400 ml cold water may be drunk in 10–15 seconds, or it may take 10 minutes, more commonly 1–4 minutes. Food is also obstructed but will slowly pass through and although it may take an hour, a whole meal can be eaten. The onset of dysphagia for liquids and solids is frequently simultaneous.

The patient with a neoplastic stricture first notices progressive obstruction to solids, then to liquids. By the time drinking is slowed it is almost impossible to get food through because if the closure by neoplasm is tight enough to stop liquids it is very much tighter against solids. Therefore only a few, if any, mouthfuls of food are attempted. Neoplasm causes a sudden and rapid progression of dysphagia over a few weeks or months which is unusual in achalasia. The pattern of symptoms overall is more useful than either radiology or endoscopy, both of which not uncommonly fail to define the neoplasm and call the obstruction achalasia.

RADIOLOGICAL EXAMINATION

The symptom pattern will nearly always define the cause of dysphagia [1]. It is possible to devise a radiological examination which will accurately define motor abnormalities, and strictures, distinguishing between benign and malignant in all but a few per cent. The essential feature is to tip the patient 10° head down and record the transport of barium uphill on video tape. The peristaltic wave may be defined and its amplitude, capacity to form a gas and liquid tight closure, and length, quantitated. The difference in motility of the wall between achalasia and systemic sclerosis is easily seen. The compliance of the wall of the body of the oesophagus is recorded while the patient drinks barium through a bent straw in the 10° head down position. The flaccidity of the wall, except where the peristaltic wave is present (and this is inhibited by repeated swallowing), allows full distension. This is even better shown if there is reflux of barium from the stomach at the same time. Any zone of increased resistance to stretch is clearly defined provided the wall is distended proximally and distally. The method produces a standard and maximum challenge and gives repeatable results. If the lumen is not adequately distended the stricture may easily be missed because it opens as easily as the adjacent normal wall until the critical circumference is reached. The diameter of the lumen of the stricture to liquid barium, defined in this way, is the same as that defined by bread soaked in barium. If barium tablets whose diameter increases in steps of 1 mm are given, the diameter of the largest tablet that can be pushed through with a drink is usually about 1 mm greater than the barium/bread diameter. When in doubt about the presence or site of an effective obstruction to food, barium tablets are given in increasing size up to 15 mm. Few people complain of dysphagia at 12 mm, rarely if at all at 15 mm bore.

The activity of the cardiac sphincter is examined first in the 10° head down antigravity position. In achalasia, or pseudoachalasia from submucosal neoplasm or post-vagotomy perioesophagitis or sometimes in post-hiatal repair dysphagia, the narrowing is seen as the barium approaches the stomach. The length, diameter and shape of the narrow zone can be quantitated. In systemic sclerosis the sphincter disappears and the channel to the stomach is not constricted. The patient then stands erect and swallows a bolus of barium. How much the oesophagogastric junction opens, the normal is 10 mm, is recorded, and the effect on the sphincter, or closed segment, of a dry swallow. Relaxation of the sphincter can be quantitated. In order to measure lengths accurately a reference is necessary, e.g. a 2 cm wire grid attached to the surface of the X-ray table. The shadow of the grid is magnified about 5% more than the barium shadow, which is magnified about 1.75–2.0 times on the radiographic film.

DISTURBANCES OF CONTRACTION AND RELAXATION

'Obstructive spasm'

'Spasm' is a word which should no longer be used. There is no good evidence of any condition in the oesophagus where persistent abnormal contraction is a cause of dysphagia, except the failure of reflex relaxation of the cardiac sphincter in achalasia and so-called 'diffuse oesophageal spasm'. The rings of contraction seen on a radiographic film in 'corkscrew' oesophagus and 'diffuse spasm' are neither persistent in time nor place but represent a writhing of the wall which is easily seen by endoscopy or radiology. The increased resistance to stretch of the wall in peptic oseophagitis and stricture is not muscle spasm because the muscle contracts and relaxes normally, but is a result of the change in physical elastic properties of the wall caused by inflammation and fibroblasts (see below). A Schatzski ring is not a muscle contraction but an elastic increased resistance to stretch at the squamo-columnar junction. If there is evidence of bolus obstruction, look for a continuous cause. Variable dysphagia is variable bolus size, not 'spasm' or nervous tension.

There are two mechanical situations which must not be confused with 'spasm'. In achalasia a grossly or moderately dilated oesophagus may have its lumen suddenly reduced to a tiny punctum by the combined effect of the cardiac sphincter and the surrounding hiatus of the diaphragm. If a square-ended endoscope is pushed towards this the flaccid lower part of the oesophageal wall immediately proximal to the sphincter flattens out over the closed hiatus and diaphragm. Consequently there may be some resistance to pushing the endoscope through. By contrast, a bougie or taper-ended endoscope pointed at the punctum will slip through without any obvious resistance to stretch. It is not spasm of the sphincter but the mechanical problem which hinders the instrument. Ability to gauge the resistance to stretch precisely is an essential part of the differential diagnosis of achalasia and submucosal neoplasm (see below).

The other similar cause of obstruction is the cricopharyngeus which is a band of striated muscle attached to either side of the cricoid cartilage, encircling and gently compressing the pharyngo-oesophageal junction to a slit. The muscle is tonically contracted by a steady stream of impulses from the medulla, relaxing momentarily when the stream is interrupted during the swallowing sequence. The normal muscle has an extraordinary compliance and lack of elastance over the normal range, for example, it will stretch abruptly from its contracted state length of 12 mm to 50 mm when a bolus passes through. Even when contracted, it has only slight resistance to stretch so that a bougie or taper-ended endoscope may be passed easily without a sense of resistance. Nevertheless, the normal cricopharyngeus often seems to offer an obstruction to a square-ended endoscope, especially if the base of the tongue and with it the hyoid and thyroid cartilages are pulled forwards. The cricopharyngeus then becomes a posterior bar across the floor of the pharynx immediately behind the cricoid cartilage. Pressure on the muscle tends to push it down rather than backwards. This again is not a problem of 'spasm' but of mechanics. Sometimes, however, the muscle is diseased and fibrosed, resisting stretch by a tapered bougie. Submucosal fibrosis which is circumferential and unrelated to fibrosis of the cricopharyngeus may also obstruct a bougie or an endoscope (see below) but neither of these are 'spasm' of the muscle.

The important concept illustrated by these examples is that normal basal tone of the fully contracted muscle of the upper and lower oesophageal sphincters does not offer palpable resistance to stretch up to 50 mm circumference (50F), nor does that of the achalasic sphincter, although it severely obstructs the passage of food and drink.

'Spasm pain'

'Spasm' as a cause of pain is still not proven. The pain associated with bolus obstruction seems to come from mucosal and not muscle receptors. The pain of heartburn is unchanged when the oesophageal muscle is pharmacologically inhibited and incapable of contraction. The spontaneous pain of achalasia and so-called symptomatic diffuse oesophageal spasm is certainly not caused by reflux and is rarely, if ever, relieved by octyl nitrite, glyceryl trinitrate or nifedipine. Violent chaotic muscular contractions are present in the wall of the achalasic oesophagus most of the time but the pain is only occasional, spontaneous, and unrelated to eating or drinking. During the pain, the patient may drink and eat without more difficulty than usual, both before and after an effective cardiomyotomy. The latter does not stop the pain, although it frequently reduces the frequency and severity.

Chest pain not caused by refluxing gastric contents stimulating the oesophageal squamous mucosa, or by myocardial ischaemia, or definable lesions of the chest wall, or cervical spondylosis, has for long been attributed to the oesophagus. The reason seems to be partly because the area of distribution of oesophageal pain is wide enough to encompass most pains; partly because severe spontaneous pain which spreads over the chest, neck and arms is known to occur in achalasia and its variant 'diffuse spasm'; and partly because no-one has found or suggested another source. Nevertheless, with rare exceptions, what I prefer to call 'non-specific chest pain' has not been shown to arise in the oesophagus. 'Painful peristalsis', 'symptomatic oesophageal peristalsis', was first described by Pope in 1976 [2], and Brand et al. [3] as 'super-peristalsis', that is, high amplitude peristaltic waves which were demonstrated by manometry and associated with angina-like pain, in patients with normal coronary angiograms. Provocation of these contractions and the pain has been described following the injection of ergometrine by Dart and colleagues [4]. The provocation test is not without hazard to the coronary arteries and myocardium; the equipment for the test is not generally available, nor the expertise required to interpret the tracings with sufficient confidence and accuracy to make a clear diagnosis.

Endoscopy and radiology are unhelpful because the appearances are normal. Treatment is empirical and frequently ineffective, namely glyceryl trinitrite tablets or nifedipine liquid under the tongue. I have seen patients in whom the pain waxed and waned like a colic, and who had discomfort or dysphagia when trying to drink during an attack of pain. Oesophageal motility was normal by radiology when pain was absent. These few patients may have had 'painful peristalsis' but scores of other patients with 'non-specific chest pain' have pain which is largely steady in intensity for minutes or hours, is unaffected by, and does not affect, eating or drinking, and is not helped by glyceryl trinitrite. It remains a mystery and I see no reason to attribute it to the oesophagus.

DISTURBANCES OF NERVE SUPPLY

Neurological disorders such as Parkinsonism, multiple system disease, cerebrovascular accidents, may disturb the propagation of the peristaltic wave into the oesophagus, or the amplitude of the peristaltic wave, and the basal tone of the sphincter. In old age the oesophagus may dilate and peristaltic amplitude decrease or disappear. Dystrophia myotonica affects smooth as well as striated muscle, with a low tone in the cricopharyngeus and a dilated almost immobile oesophagus. Disorganized contractions or loss of peristalsis and reduction in tone of the cardiac sphincter are sometimes seen in diabetic and in alcoholic autonomic neuropathy. None of these changes, however, produce symptoms.

The lesion in achalasia, and almost certainly in symptomatic diffuse oesophageal spasm, is loss of the post-ganglionic neurone and its associated cholinesterase. Destruction of these neurones is not an all or none process, and is not necessarily progressive or continuing. At any one time the capacity for peristalsis will depend on how many post-ganglionic neurones are left in Auerbach's plexus in the body of the oesophagus; and the capacity to relax the cardiac sphincter from its basal tonic state will depend on the proportion of post-ganglionic cells left in the sphincter. The basal tone of the sphincter is up to two times greater than normal, perhaps because of loss of local cholinesterase. This increase in tone plus the failure to relax is enough to resist the opening force of a column of water 22 cm high plus the contraction of part of the wall, so that the lumen of the sphincter is seen by radiology to be stretched to 1–4 mm at best, while the patient is eating or drinking. There is no obstruction to a bougie. In 'diffuse spasm' there may be some recognizable remnants of the peristaltic wave and partial relaxation of the sphincter with a swallow. Spontaneous pain occurs equally in both diffuse spasm and achalasia. The differences in other symptoms, in the motor activity of the wall and sphincter, are a matter of degree and in a personal consecutive series of more than 500 patients I have not found a useful or meaningful dividing line between achalasia and diffuse spasm. The distinction is largely based on manometric estimates of wall and sphincter activity leading to a man-made distinction based on tracings and not on pathology. If the patient has dysphagia, a cardiomyotomy relieves the dysphagia. There is no need for the myotomy to extend beyond the sphincter and 1 cm proximal to it. Pain is not cured by extending the myotomy, but a mucosal epiphrenic diverticulum is produced which itself can be a cause of post-myotomy dysphagia. The response to the mecholyl test seems to depend on what proportion of the post-ganglionic neurones and their associated cholinesterase survives. The greater the loss of neurones the greater the mecholyl response.

After the removal of the obstruction caused by the sphincter by a cardiomyotomy, the body of the oesophagus usually becomes much narrower and the amount of persisting peristaltic activity is much more easily determined by radiology. Many a large achalasic oesophagus turns into an active 'diffuse spasm-like' gullet which can propel barium into the stomach, almost emptying itself when the patient is in the 10° head down position. These motor changes are easy to see by radiology, but difficult to see at endoscopy, and impossible to feel. Manometry is not necessary for the diagnosis.

MUSCLE DISEASE

In polymyositis, dermatomyositis, scleroderma and systemic sclerosis there is a loss of striated, cardiac and smooth muscle to varying degrees. Smooth muscle is sometimes lost in systemic lupus. The loss of smooth muscle in the oesophagus results in weakness and eventual failure of the peristaltic wave and flaccid distension of the body. The sphincter disappears and the wall stretches leaving the lumen open except for the section closed by the hiatus of the diaphragm. These changes do not usually cause dysphagia. If the muscle walls of the hiatus decrease in strength and amount the antireflux mechanism fails and reflux oesophagitis is likely to follow, then a peptic stricture. These strictures are characteristically wide bore, e.g. 8–12 mm and are recognizable radiographically because the lumen is constant in size throughout a swallowing sequence. The stricture obstructs solid food but may be compliant enough to allow the oesophagoscope to pass easily. The lack of motor activity is usually easily seen; the mucosa looks normal except when oesophagitis develops, because the disease does not involve mucous membranes. The stricture is usually missed because it is too compliant to feel.

CHANGES IN COMPLIANCE AND ELASTANCE

The two physical properties of compliance and elastance are of crucial importance in the production of symptoms of dysphagia and in its management. *Compliance* is the ease with which the wall can be stretched, that is, it is inversely proportional to the resistance to stretch. The wall of the body of the oesophagus is flaccid except when a peristaltic wave is passing through and has a very high compliance, capable of changing from 15 mm circumference to 60 mm in a fraction of a second during aerophagy for example. The relaxed cardiac sphincter is almost equally compliant, the contracted normal sphincter is a little less so, and the achalasic sphincter a little less compliant still. The resistance to stretch depends on smooth muscle contraction, however, which is easily overcome by a bougie or tapered endoscope, but not by swallowed food and drink. Changes in the composition of the wall in mucosal oesophagitis, which often extends over many centimetres, do not alter compliance in a way which we can detect by radiology, although sometimes the patient seems to be aware of it through the sensation that a bolus is being pushed through a tender zone. The highly localized submucosal changes associated with stricture formation cause a loss of compliance which is only a few millimetres long, with an abrupt change from one compliance to another, resulting in easy opening to 2–12 mm diameter (6–40 mm circumference) only. These two types of compliance are characteristic but unexplained. Of 404 consecutive benign strictures, 52% were less than 5 mm, 23% were 5–10 mm long. Malignant strictures are much longer and there is no sharp change in compliance at the end of the constriction.

Benign peptic strictures illustrate the complexity of the behaviour of the wall. At least two thirds of peptic strictures are within the sphincter segment, which is about 18 mm long. The whole sphincter including the stricture, closes normally with a basal tone in the normal range, but when relaxed and challenged by a descending bolus the 'stricture' will stretch to 2–12 mm diameter, but the adjacent sphincter fibres stretch to 15–20 mm. If the stricture is in the body of the oesophagus, the stricture is closed by the peristaltic wave and a subsequent bolus stretches the adjacent wall to 15–25 mm. These measurements are consistent from one week to another and are independent of the amount of oesophagitis. The stricture is therefore *not* caused by muscle contraction but by a change in the physical properties of the tissue, which does not seem to manifest itself until a certain diameter of lumen is reached. This diameter is almost the same whether the bolus is liquid or solid.

Elastance is the force tending to return the wall to its original length after it has been stretched. A 3 mm hole in a sheet of paper (which has no elastance in this context) may be enlarged by pushing a finger through it, and so may a 3 mm hole in a sheet of rubber, which has elastance. Different kinds and thicknesses of rubber will have difference elastances although they might have a similar compliance. All obstructions in the pharynx, oesophagus and hiatus have some elastance.

To reduce elastance, the tissue must be disrupted in some way. The achalasic sphincter has to be stretched to 45 mm diameter (140 mm circumference) to make much impression on the dysphagia, because the sphincter is normal smooth muscle. The hiatus is muscular and equally compliant and elastic (it too is stretched to 140 mm circumference when the achalasic sphincter is dilated) so that to increase the compliance (i.e. reduce the elastance) when the hiatus has been sewn up too tight at a hiatal repair, the muscle fibres must be torn or the stitch torn out. It is not surprising that conventional bouginage has little useful effect.

Peptic strictures behave differently and unpredictably. A compliant stricture may have little elastance and open widely for months after a single dilatation, or may be so elastic that the next day the lumen is the same as before the dilatation. In 31 dilatations of peptic strictures to a mean circumference of 43 mm (43 FG) the mean predilatation circumference to food was 19 mm and the mean post-dilatation circumference was 21 mm. Nevertheless, with each successive dilatation some elastance is usually lost. Healing of oesophagitis and re-epithelialization does not always alter the compliance and elastance of the underlying wall, but persistence of the inflammatory process certainly perpetuates the loss of compliance.

The loss of compliance caused by myopathy and fibrosis of the cricopharyngeus muscle, or by submucosal fibrosis of the pharyngo-oesophageal junction, or post-vagotomy perioesophagitis with fibrosis also varies from slight to severe. The elastance is unpredictable but usually diminishes with each successive dilatation. Neoplasm whether luminal, or submucosal and invisible, or extra-oesophageal has a virtually irreducible elastance. The compliance is variable from something which an endoscope can scarcely feel, to impenetrability.

THE ROLES OF ENDOSCOPY AND RADIOLOGY

Endoscopy frequently changes the diameter and shape of the lumen of some kinds of obstruction temporarily. For this reason alone it is preferable to carry out the radiological examination of the oesophagus before endoscopy. In addition, good radiology can identify the position and often the nature of lesions, which are then more effectively examined in detail by endoscopy. The essential importance of the 'feel' with the endoscope in the differential diagnosis of lesions which close the lumen to liquids is exemplified by the difference between the compliant gentle closure of achalasia and the tight closure of encircling neoplasm, which may be impossible to distinguish with certainty by radiology. Good radiology will demonstrate the type and cause of a patient's symptoms with great accuracy and precision.

REFERENCES

1. Edwards, D. A. W. (1976) Discriminatory value of symptoms in the differential diagnosis of dysphagia. *Clin. Gastroenterol.*, **5** (**No. 1**), 49–57.
2. Pope C. E. (1976) Abnormalities of peristaltic amplitude and force – a clue to the aetiology of chest pain. In *Proceedings of the Fifth International Symposium on Gastrointestinal Motility* (ed. G. Vantrappen), Typoff-Press, Herentals, pp. 380–6.
3. Brand, D. L., Martin, D. and Pope, C. E. (1977) Oesophageal manometrics in patients with angina-like chest pain. *Dig. Dis.*, **22**, 300–4.
4. Dart, A. M., Alban-Davies, H., Lowndes, R., Dalal, J. J., Ruttley, M. S. T. and Henderson, A. H. (1980) Oesophageal spasm and 'angina': diagnostic value of ergometrine provocation. *Eur. Heart J.*, **1**, 91–5.

13

The problem of diagnosing reflux

D. A. W. EDWARDS

Most of us are practising clinicians faced with a patient with certain symptoms or signs. We want to know the cause of the symptoms and how vigorously to treat them. We can approach this problem by saying either 'what is the *necessary* information on which to make these decisions' or 'how many tests can I do that might tell me something about what is happening', and we might even add 'because it would be interesting to do them all'. The first is the most cost-effective approach – the second is perhaps the more intellectually stimulating, although it has three main disadvantages apart from wasting time and money. They are: (a) giving the wrong or misleading information, (b) repeating the same information, and (c) adding confusion.

(a) By 'giving the wrong or misleading information' in the context of reflux, I mean for example, that a test which demonstrates that reflux occurs does not answer the clinician's question about whether the patient's symptoms are *caused* by reflux, or how vigorously should he treat the reflux (see below).

(b) By 'repeating the same information' I mean that a new test may be just another way of showing the same phenomenon, for example the scintiscan test for reflux demonstrates what barium can demonstrate because the isotope-labelled liquid behaves as barium behaves, and the pH electrode is recording almost the same thing.

(c) By 'adding confusion' I mean that doing more tests does not make an action decision any easier nor reduce error. If we do a test (A), we get a 'yes' (Y), 'no' (N) or 'don't know or can't decide' (DK) answer. There are 3 action decisions: treat (T); not treat (NT); and think again (X). If we do another test (B), the answers may be the same or different, but there is a possibility that there will be a 3^2 combination of results and 3^2 action decisions to make (see Table 13.1).

Table 13.1 Results of tests

Test A	Y	Y	Y	N	N	N	DK	DK	DK
Test B	Y	N	DK	Y	N	DK	Y	N	DK
Actions to be decided	T	?	?	?	NT	?	?	?	?

If the test gives 3 possible results (Y, N, DK), the number of possible combinations of results, and decisions to be made, will be 3 to the power of the number of different tests carried out, e.g. 3^n. But, there are only 3 decisions or actions, namely (a) the diagnosis is (A) or treat; (b) the diagnosis is not (A) or not treat; (c) the diagnosis or need to treat is uncertain. Decisions are usually made on the results of only one or two tests, and it is intellectually and financially inefficient to do a test if the result is not going to modify an action decision based upon another test result already obtained. We should choose, as far as possible, tests whose answers cannot be overridden, that is tests which discriminate rather than simply provide interesting information. 'Cannot' in the last sentence may seem too strong a word, and if it means a probability of 0, it is too strong. We have to decide on the basis of time, money and resources how often we think we should carry out a test which has a 1 in 20 or 1 in 100 or 1 in 1000 or 1 in 10 000 chance of changing a diagnosis or treatment decision. Such a decision often needs to be made about, for example, endoscopy. Given a set of symptoms and a certain radiological appearance, what is the probability that endoscopy will come up with an answer that is as good as or better? This probability will unfortunately depend on who took the history, how well the doctor and patient were communicating, how good the radiologist was and how well he was briefed, and how good or experienced the endoscopist was. The same limitations apply equally to manometry, pH recording and scintiscans. It is a measure of our shame and our incompetence sometimes that we feel we have to do another test because we know that the local error rate is high [1]. Before 'doing a test' we should decide what we are going to do with the answer and how its combination with the results of other tests will produce an action decision. In other words, we still have to decide which answer to act upon when we get conflicting information.

Gastro-oesophageal reflux provides many illustrations of this philosophy. Different tests record different variables, have high false negative rates and various false positive rates, and often provide information that is irrelevant. Why are we concerned about reflux? Because it sometimes produces symptoms and occasionally produces complications? Why are we concerned about the symptoms? Because they include chest pain which might be an indication of impending death from myocardial ischaemia or 'dysphagia' which might be caused by cancer, or because recurrent bronchopneumonia or pulmonary fibrosis is sometimes caused by aspiration of regurgitated oesophageal contents? Do we wish to know whether surgery is likely to be the best treatment? Each question is usually best answered by a different investigation. For example, 'are the patient's symptoms caused by reflux?' is best answered by the pattern of symptoms. 'Has the patient the capacity to herniate stomach or for abnormal reflux?' is best answered by radiology. 'Does the patient have abnormal reflux during some or all of their daily and nightly activities?' is best answered by 24 hour pH monitoring. 'Does the patient ever suffer from this reflux?' can only be answered by this method. 'Is surgery likely to make much difference?' is best answered by assessment of the size of the hiatus and the ease of hiatal flow by radiology.

Part of the problem about not knowing what to do about reflux arises from a lack of understanding of the mechanisms of reflux, part from the confusion about what is a relevant question to ask and part from the confusion about which question a particular test can answer. This chapter discusses some of these points in detail.

NORMAL AND ABNORMAL REFLUX AND THE ANTIREFLUX MECHANISM

All normal people reflux regularly after meals. This normal, physiological reflux, which is small in volume, seems to be caused by an increase in intragastric pressure produced by contraction of the stomach wall, which overcomes whatever squeeze the cardiac sphincter has at the time. Increasing intra-abdominal pressure or change of posture does not induce it, nor does relaxing the sphincter by swallowing. Sometimes it is so marked that the refluxate reaches the mouth when the subject is standing or sitting. This has been called rumination and it seems to be an exaggeration of normal physiological reflux. It probably includes some of what are called 'upright refluxers'. Barium seems to inhibit the phenomenon since it is not seen radiologically. It is rare, if it has been recorded, during a scintiscan. It is clearly demonstrated by a pH electrode in the oesophagus [2]. The cardiac sphincter seems to protect the oesophagus from changes in *intragastric* pressure produced by contraction of the *stomach* wall. By contrast, the hiatal mechanism seems to protect the oesophagus from changes in *intra-abdominal* pressure produced by contraction of the abdominal wall. It seems to protect in 3 ways:

(a) By contraction of the diaphragmatic hiatus upon the oesophagus or herniated stomach passing through it with a compressing force normally greater than intra-abdominal pressure.

(b) By preserving a section of the cardiac sphincter within the abdomen so that the sphincter is compressed by intra-abdominal pressure as much as the stomach is, thereby eliminating any challenge to the sphincter from increasing intra-abdominal pressure.

(c) By creating a 'flutter valve' condition at the hiatus from the tube of gut passing through a slit so that the greater the difference in pressure between abdomen and thorax, the more firmly is the tube closed.

Failure of this hiatal mechanism allows the sphincter to be challenged by the difference in pressure between abdomen and thorax. This difference is increased during sobbing, during the inspiratory phase preceding a cough, or increasing intra-abdominal pressure. Herniation of the sphincter and some stomach does not always mean that the sphincter will be challenged by intra-abdominal pressure because the hiatus may still be snug enough to compress the tube of stomach, or to form the flutter valve with it. The challenge to the sphincter will depend upon the ease of hiatal flow of gastric contents from abdominal to thoracic stomach. The size and shape of the hiatus change with body position and movement so that the ease and amount of hiatal flow also change. Breakdown of this component of the antireflux mechanism is associated with what may be called abnormal reflux. This kind of reflux may be demonstrated radiologically in certain positions but not necessarily in all, for example, it may occur when bending with a full stomach, but not when lying down or when the stomach is not so full. It most commonly occurs during the movement of rolling from the left side onto the back or the back onto the right side, and least commonly when rolling onto the left side. The patient knows which side, position or movement is most likely to provoke symptoms and they should be examined in that way. This phenomenon explains why different methods of testing for reflux may give different answers.

Relative competence or incompetence of the hiatus is what determines the severity of abnormal reflux and this is how surgery helps – by reducing the size of the hiatus rather than the size of the hernia. The probability that surgery will permanently stop abnormal hiatal flow is 1:2 to 1:5 and if symptoms are bad because of a very sensitive mucosa rather than severe hiatal flow, surgery has a poor chance of success. The demonstration of the capacity to herniate the sphincter and some stomach under the reasonable stresses of daily life means the capacity for abnormal reflux is present but does not mean that it occurs frequently or causes suffering. Patients capable of abnormal reflux are entitled to have as much normal physiological reflux as normal subjects. How can we distinguish between physiological and abnormal reflux and is it worthwhile to do so? [3].

SYMPTOMS

Before discussing methods, it is important to consider the relationship between reflux and symptoms. We all have physiological reflux but most of us get symptoms from it only rarely, or only after certain food or drink. Most of the time most patients with the capacity for abnormal reflux do not get symptoms, and when they do, these symptoms can be considerably reduced by medications which do not reduce the volume or frequency of reflux, but do reduce the corrosiveness of the refluxate. Moreover, there is good evidence that the sensitivity of the oesophageal squamous epithelium is at least as important a variable in the production of symptoms as is the corrosiveness of the refluxate. It seems to change from time to time in the same person, and probably increases in vulnerability with age. Symptoms of the hiatal–hernia reflux syndrome do not come from the herniation nor the process of herniation; occasionally they may possibly arise from the herniated gastric mucosa. Their essential features are gastric contents in the mouth, which is a mechanical effect, and irritation or damage to the squamous epithelium, which is a corrosive effect depending on an equilibrium between corrosiveness, repair and sensitivity [4].

Possible conditions

If we set up a table of the possible combinations of physiological reflux, hiatal herniation with abnormal reflux, symptoms and oesophagitis we find it is possible to have physiological reflux with or without symptoms and with or without oesophagitis (however defined, although histological oesophagitis is uncommon with physiological reflux); to have the capacity to herniate stomach with or without abnormal reflux; and to have abnormal reflux with or without symptoms and with or without oesophagitis. All these combinations are common in clinical practice.

Diagnosis or quantitation

What, then, do we want to know, and why? Is it important simply to know that a person can reflux? or that they have a hiatal hernia? When a patient presents with symptoms, it is the symptoms themselves that determine their cause in this context. The detection of reflux by pH electrode or scintiscan; or of the capacity to herniate stomach by endoscopy or barium or scintiscan, cannot by itself tell us whether the symptoms of which the patient complains are caused by the reflux or hernia because these phenomena are so commonly asymptomatic. The only useful tests for the cause of symptoms are:

(a) The nature and pattern of the symptoms themselves
(b) A test which provokes the symptom
(c) A device which records symptoms and reflux simultaneously
(d) A test which identifies a pathological specific consequence of reflux e.g. endoscopy and biopsy

Circumstantial evidence must sometimes be admitted. One of the causes of chronic lung disease is aspiration of regurgitated gastric contents. The demonstration of gross reflux and regurgitation in that patient would be strong circumstantial evidence of association. The demonstration of abnormal reflux in a patient with a stricture at the squamocolumnar junction would be reasonable circumstantial evidence in favour of the stricture being peptic, and if *abnormal* reflux could not be demonstrated, the nature of the stricture would be in doubt. If a stricture is *not* at the squamocolumnar junction its association with reflux is almost certainly fortuitous.

Quantitation

Quantitation of reflux may be important once we have decided that the symptoms are caused by reflux. For example, if the breakdown of the mechanical part of the antireflux mechanism (the hiatal factor) is severe, pharmacological measures will fail and only mechanical measures including surgery are likely to help, although there is no guarantee they will succeed. Most patients with abnormal reflux have a mild to moderate amount which is usually amenable to medical measures. Sometimes the oesophageal mucosa is so sensitivie that even small amounts of reflux cause great distress. Most clinicians match the severity of treatment to the severity of symptoms and quantitation of reflux does not always give the answer appropriate to the symptoms. The urge to measure for measurement's sake is sound philosophy if one is measuring the right variable and can use the answer in a useful calculation. Symptoms are difficult to measure.

METHODS OF DETECTION AND QUANTITATION

Radiology

Few physicians are brave enough to make a firm diagnosis of reflux on symptoms alone, although it is possible to do so. Most would require a barium examination, partly because they think (wrongly) that the demonstration of herniation or reflux provides the answer (it only provides spurious comfort to the doctor) and partly to exclude anything else. Radiology can show the capacity to herniate stomach and reflux barium when the antireflux mechanism is challenged by the difference between intra-abdominal and intrathoracic pressure. It can quantitate the size of the loculus and the severity of the mechanical problem by estimating the size of the hiatus and the ease of hiatal flow of contents across it. It can quantitate the quality of the peristaltic wave and its capacity to clear contents into the stomach against a challenge of reflux better than manometry or pH electrode (see below). It can identify a stricture and sometimes demonstrate ulcerating oesophagitis. It can recognize gall stones, peptic ulcer of the stomach and duodenum, and other lesions. It cannot say if the symptoms are caused by reflux and it cannot detect or quantitate normal physiological reflux [3]. The disadvantages of radiology are that (a) the method of examination is not standardized and variations in technique influence the answers obtained, and (b) digitization and therefore communication of results is not as convenient as with scintiscan or pH electrode. The development of the latter methods has been fostered by the clinician's dissatisfaction with the information that radiologists have provided, as well as his lack of understanding of what radiology can and cannot do. There is also an element of mystique as well as certainty about computer printouts of densities and areas and of pH changes, that radiographic films lack. Radiology will remain, with endoscopy, the first line of investigation. It would seem sensible to attempt to improve the quality and quantity of information it provides as a routine, leaving 24 hour-pH monitoring for specific research projects and perhaps as a supra-regional service for the difficult problem.

pH monitoring and recording

Miniature glass electrodes suitable for swallowing became commercially available in the 1950s and a telemetering 'radiopill' soon followed. The glass electrode was uncomfortably large to pass through the nose and very susceptible to scratching. The pH radiopill had an antimony electrode and was plagued by electronic problems. In recent years, the glass electrode has been miniaturized and the British pH radiopill has become a robust electronically stable glass electrode [5]. Both types of sensor now record on tape on portable cassette recorders with channels for event recording such as the position of the patient or whether they felt a symptom. They are worn at home during normal waking and sleeping activity. Some models are commercially available [6]. Computer programs are available for various methods of analysis of the records which eliminate observer variation. Vantrappen and colleagues [7] record pH from two glass electrodes and an intraluminal reference electrode, and pressure from three intergrated-sensor type transducers. The cassette recorder contains pH and pressure amplifiers, modulators for pH, pressure signals and 4 track tape for 24 hours. Time multiplexing allows signals from two pH electrodes, an event marker for the patient and two marker channels for the operator to record on one channel, with pressures on the other three. By extending the recording period over 24 hours and by allowing the patient to move freely and live a normal daily routine, it is possible to demonstrate episodes of reflux and any association with symptoms that are more relevant to normal life than the postures of radiology or scintigraphy or endoscopy. The system allows visual replay on a paper recorder and computated and automated analyses and quantitation of a large number of variables.

They confirmed Pattrick's original observations [2] that healthy 'non-refluxers' very rarely have episodes of reflux during the night, lying down, but have daily episodes of reflux with the intra-oesophageal electrode recording a pH of less than 4, 1–5% of the time. They also demonstrated reflux when subjects were sitting and standing, confirming what we have all experienced ourselves; and frequent prolonged episodes of low pH at the surface of the electrode in a supine patient with oesophagitis. They had no problem in recording frequent and prolonged changes of pH at the electrode in patients with pathological changes of the mucosa, but they agree that the definition of normality is difficult. Branicki *et al.* [5] use a radiopill glass electrode anchored in the oesophagus by a thread taped to the cheek with a portable receiver and tape recorder. One potential advantage of portable 24 hour monitoring is the ability to classify patients into upright refluxers, supine refluxers and combined upright and supine refluxers (see also Johnson and De Meester [8]). All three groups may have heartburn, but the difference may be important for prognosis and treatment. Several investigators have found, for example, that upright refluxers rarely develop oesophagitis, which is more frequent in supine refluxers, and most severe in combined refluxers. It can be argued that the patient or the radiologist or a combination of both can separate the groups almost as well.

So far, research workers in this field have compared the results obtained on normal asymptomatic subjects with those obtained in patients with endoscopically proven oesophagitis. This method *highlights* the differences, and shows that these can be recorded. We are not, however, looking for a test that agrees with what we know already. Instead, we are looking for a procedure which, when applied to patients who are suffering and who are *without* a diagnosis, will tell us precisely *why* they are suffering. Vantrappen *et al.* [7] applied a discriminant function analysis to records from normals and from those with severe oesophagitis. The best discriminant was the number of reflux episodes lasting longer than 5 minutes in the 24 hour period; the next best was the number of similar episodes occurring in the night; and the next best was the same variable in the postprandial period. The number of reflux episodes (unqualified) was not helpful. It remains to be seen with what accuracy these or other discriminants will identify management categories for the next 200 patients who attend each of our clinics with symptoms suggestive of reflux.

As a research tool for determining the pattern of reflux in everyday life in apparently normal people and of sufferers before and after a specific treatment, the portable 24 hour pH monitoring device seems to have considerable potential. The anchored radiopill, with only a thread through the mouth, is probably more comfortable for the patient than the standard pH electrode assembly. Two major problems still have to be solved, (a) how to read and score the record, and (b) how to interpret longer episodes on the record of low pH. Scoring is commonly by (1) the number of low pH episodes during 24 hours, (2) how long the pH is less than 4 in the 24 hours, (3) how long each episode is of less than pH 4 on the record. It seems likely that there will be considerable overlap in the distribution of values of these variables between people with and those without symptoms.

The most important part of the analysis seems likely to be the association between change of pH and the recording of the complained-of symptoms. Some symptoms such as cough or wheezing may precede a reflux episode; many reflux episodes pass without notice by the patient. De Meester and colleagues [9] have a keyboard of common symptoms for the patient to punch. Vantrappen and colleagues [7] record both pH and pressure with symptoms and events. The pH electrode records the concentration of $(H)^+$ at the surface of the electrode, it does not measure the total quantity of $(H)^+$ in the oesophagus. It is therefore unsuitable for measuring the amount of reflux. There is a marked discrepancy between the ability of a peristaltic wave to clear visible barium from the oesophagus and to clear hydrogen ions from the glass electrode. In many thousands of barium examinations of the hiatal hernia reflux syndrome, I have watched a single peristaltic wave sweep a bolus of barium uphill into the stomach, leaving little or nothing visible behind. Occasionally, the clearing is not so good, especially if the patient swallows repeatedly, which inhibits the propagation of the wave. After an episode of abnormal reflux however, recorded by a pH electrode, it is usual to find that many swallows are necessary before the pH of the surface of the glass electrode is above 4. Where are these hydrions hiding? In the mucus adherent to the electrode or in the mucus layer on the mucosa, or in the eroded mucosa? What is clear is that the persistence of a pH of less than 4 on the surface of the electrode does not mean that the gullet is flooded with gastric contents, or that the oesophageal clearing process is impaired, or that a 'reflux episode' lasts continuously for minutes or hours. It must also be remembered that when the patient is standing or sitting, most of the herniation is reduced into the abdomen. If the electrode is placed just above the sphincter in this position, when the patient lies down the herniation may increase, and the sphincter rides up over the electrode, which is then in the stomach. Apart from this difficulty, prolonged mobile pH recording is probably the most objective tool in the quantiative assessment of reflux, but it only quantitates – it doesn't explain whether symptoms are caused by reflux, unless there is a repeated and consistent coincidence of symptoms and reflux.

Endoscopy

Endoscopy is not an appropriate *diagnostic* tool in the investigation of reflux symptoms or chest pain. It recognizes and may help to quantitate damage to the squamous epithelium, but it does not recognize either irritation or sensitivity or symptoms. It is not as specific or sensitive as good radiology in detecting benign or malignant strictures (see Chapter 12).

It is often said that every patient with symptoms associated with the oesophagus should have an endoscopy to exclude cancer. The incidence of diagnosing cancer of the oesophagus in the absence of symptoms or radiological abnormality of the oesophagus is extremely low in Great Britain although it may be greater in other countries. The incidence of unsuspected cancer or other lesion in the stomach as a cause of vague symptoms is higher. The disadvantages of endoscopy are:

(a) If nothing abnormal is seen, there is the possibility of a tendency for the clinician to consider that the patient is making an undue fuss, even when the symptoms indicate a condition that is not commonly clearly defined by endoscopy.

(b) The cost/benefit ratio is much too high for a primary procedure.

(c) Patients frequently find it unpleasant and often distressing, according to their discussions with non-endoscopists.

(d) A normal endoscopy does not exclude anything, there is a high false negative rate for most common lesions.

(e) There is poor correlation between symptoms and endoscopic appearance in reflux disease, for example, the symptoms may be severe with no visible abnormality and very mild histological change, or the symptoms may be mild or uncomplained of in the presence of chronic erosive oesophagitis.

Where the final treatment decision such as whether to operate or not, rests upon the result of endoscopy, it may be justifiable in reflux disease. It seems uncommon for a major point of principle or detail in the medical management of reflux disease to be determined by endoscopy findings rather than by symptoms.

Manometry

At one time it was widely believed that the cardiac sphincter was the sole barrier to reflux of any kind, and it was equally widely believed that measuring the resting squeeze of the sphincter would identify those patients who were refluxing. The realization that this is not true is spreading and manometry has no useful place in the routine investigation of reflux. Recording sphincter squeeze may have value in a research program about reflux, and recording the pattern and amplitude of peristaltic waves in the body of the oesophagus may help in the investigation of 'non-specific chest pain'. Manometry requires smoothly running, frequently used equipment, and experienced operators who thoroughly understand the oeso- phagus and what manometry records. Even then the tracings have poor reproducibility in the same patient and may be difficult to interpret. Relative sensitivity and selectivity are too low even when other methods are badly carried out.

Scintiscanning

Scintiscanning is a recent development of nuclear medicine. The stomach is filled with a colloid containing 99^mtechnetium pertechnate, the patient lies flat under a gamma camera and the position of the radionuclide is recorded with automated quantitation. The flow of gastric contents from abdominal to herniated thoracic stomach, and from stomach to oesophagus can be recorded [10]. The radionuclide behaves in the same way as barium. The limitations on the position and movement of the patient in the gamma camera limits the scope of the search for the capacity to herniate stomach and reflux abnormally, compared with what can be achieved by barium radiography. The advantages claimed for scintiscanning are:

(a) The lower dose of ionising radiation than radiography gives (although no- one has suggested that the radiological examination be dispensed with)
(b) It is better tolerated by infants and children
(c) Quantitation is three dimensional compared with two dimensional quanti- tation of barium, and quantitation is easily digitized automatically, so removing observer error.

It is questionable whether such increased precision will alter management decisions based on other criteria which will inevitably be used. A small improvement in radiological technique should provide at least as much necessary information. When they are tolerated, both radiology and pH recording provide more information and a better coverage of daily life activity than scintiscanning when such detail is required.

Acid infusion

Acid infusion recognizes a low threshold of sensitivity of the mucosa to acid, and may stimulate or reproduce a pain or other sensation which can be compared with a symptom by the patient. The effect of acid fruit juices, hot drinks and alcohol stronger than about 8% is a simpler and cheaper test, although perhaps not so sensitive. It has the merit that it is part of the patient's symptoms. When the effect of acid infusion on hand-picked normals is compared with the effect on patients suffering from the effects of reflux, the results are encouraging. When the test is applied routinely to all patients suspected of suffering from reflux the results are often confusing and uncertain, or do not accord with the final decision.

CONCLUSIONS

The clinician with a heavy work load should remember firstly, enough is enough (symptoms ± radiology) most of the time, and when it is not, a supraregional centre is the right place for the sophisticated test that can be slightly more discriminating, because there it can be performed often enough for the equipment and its operator to produce reliable results. Secondly, a clear distinction must be made between sophisticated methods and machines which are designed and are suitable for well-planned and much needed research aimed at improving our understanding; and exciting new electronic gadgetry which produces a print out for the notes and by-passes the doctor–patient interface. Generally speaking, the patient (the symptoms) has been right more often than the clinician (who may not have communicated very well) who should have been right more often than the radiologist, who should have been right more often than the endoscopist. Manometry has had its day. Scintiscanning seems at best equal to radiology. Twenty-four hour portable pH monitoring shows promise for detecting episodes of reflux and associating them with symptoms, but has yet to prove its capacity for meaningful quantitation of reflux.

REFERENCES

1. Edwards, D. A. W. (1975) Discriminative information in the diagnosis of dysphagia. *J. R. Coll. Phys. (London)*, **9**, 257–63.
2. Pattrick, F. G. (1970) Investigation of gastrooesophageal reflux in various positions with a two lumen pH electrode. *Gut*, **11**, 659.
3. Edwards, D. A. W. (1982) The anti-reflux mechanism, its disorders and their consequences. *Clin. Gastroenterol.*, **11**, 479–96.
4. Edwards, D. A. W. (1973) Symposium on Gastrooesophageal Reflux and its complications. *Gut*, **14**, 233–7.
5. Branicki, F. J., Evans, D. F., Ogilvie, A. L. *et al.* (1982) Ambulatory monitoring of oesophageal pH in reflux oesophagitis using a portable radiotelemetry system. *Gut*, **23**, 992–8.
6. Vantrappen, G. (1983) Personal communication.
7. Vantrappen, G., Serraes, J., Janssens, H. and Peeters, T. (1982) *Twenty-four hour esophageal pH and pressure recording in out patients.* In *Motility of the Digestive Tract.* (ed. M. Weinbeck), Raven Press, New York.

8. Johnson, L. F. and De Meester, T. R. (1974) Twenty-four hour pH monitoring of the distal oesophagus. *Am. J. Gastroenterol.*, **62**, 325–32.
9. De Meester, T. R., Wang, C. I., Wernly, J. A. *et al.* (1980) Techniques, indications and clinical use of 24 hour oesophageal pH monitoring. *J. Thorac. Cardiovasc. Surg.*, **79**, 656–67.
10. Fisher, R. S., Malmud, L. S., Roberts, G. S. and Lobis, I. F. (1976) Gastrooesophageal (GE) scintiscanning to detect and quantitate GE reflux. *Gastroenterology*, **70**, 301–8.

14

Gastro-oesophageal reflux: aspects of management

L. R. CELESTIN

Gastro-oesophageal reflux is a normal physiological event occurring with a frequency and volume which are such that the normal oesophagus clears it without damage to its mucosa. The factors responsible for this physiological clearance are co-ordinated oesophageal motility and swallowing of saliva. The latter takes place at approximately two minute intervals in volumes of about 0.5 ml. During sleeping hours swallowing is totally switched off. The factor responsible for limiting reflux is a competent lower oesophageal sphincter (LOS).

A clearer understanding of this barrier has led to improved medical and surgical remedies of the state in which the physiological event becomes a pathological one, that is an event in which injury to the oesophagus occurs.

We have moved away from the obsession with an anatomical defect, namely a hiatus hernia, to the realization that it is the actual incompetence of the sphincter that determines reflux. This has been further reinforced by the fact that 50% of radiologically demonstrable hernias do not cause symptoms; while absence of a hernia does not preclude reflux. From a therapeutic point of view incompetence should be looked upon as primary or as secondary.

There can be symptoms of reflux without a hernia – primary incompetence; or a hernia without symptoms – normal competence; or a hernia with symptoms – secondary incompetence. Symptomatic treatment will alleviate the patient's complaints, while permanent cure of the reflux lies in restoring to that natural barrier its mechanical ability to prevent the undue escape of gastroduodenal juices into the oesophagus. Like all peptic disorders, reflux must be treated to a conclusion; and relapse after cessation of symptomatic or conservative treatment must be deemed a failure. The choice lies between the endless treatment of a condition, with all its inconveniences and tedium, and a quicker surgical solution with its risks and possible failures.

What then must be the rationale behind treatment?

The LOS protects two systems, the respiratory and the pharyngo-oesophageal, against two irritants, gastric acid peptic juice, and duodenal alkaline bile and pancreatic juice. When the LOS fails and one or other system is affected, symptomatic reflux results. The patient experiences the regurgitation of acid-tasting or of bitter fluid; or complains of the pulmonary complications of reflux; or may even get incarceration of the cardia into the hernia with severe pain. All these are purely *mechanical* problems requiring a mechanical solution.

The grafting of a chemical problem on to this mechanical one leads to secondary motor disorder. At first it is hypertonic, experienced as spasm – typical sudden dysphagia at the start of a meal. Later there results a patulous or hypotonic cardia with reflux oesophagitis, with its postprandial burning discomfort, a condition first reported as peptic oesophagitis in 1935 by Winkelstein [1].

Three factors lead to injury of the oesophageal mucosa and require to be dealt with:

(a) Prolonged contact of irritant with the mucosa
(b) Potency of the damaging refluxant
(c) Defence capacity of the mucosa

Contact time of irritant

Impaired LOS tone and increase in the volume of gastric contents will increase the ease of reflux thus increasing the *frequency* of contact.

Impaired oesophageal motor activity and delayed gastric emptying diminishes clearance and thus increases the *duration* of contact.

Such reflux can be reduced by the usual advice of avoiding large meals, reducing overweight and attending to postural measures – namely sleeping propped up at night and guarding during the day against bending, stooping or the wearing of tight garments. Smoking, alcohol, fat and possibly chocolate lower LOS tone and should be avoided. If pyloric hold up is present, surgery may be required.

Only one aspect of medical treatment aims at mimicking surgery – namely increasing LOS tone. Metoclopramide is a popular drug for reinforcing the sphincter, and more recently a dopamine receptor blocker, domperidone, has been suggested but its use is not without controversy. On the other hand, guaiacol in a dilution of 1:10 000 has been shown to increase sphincter tone and improve oesophageal clearing. But probably the best drug is bethanecol in doses of up to 25 mg three or four times a day. It has been shown to increase the resting LOS tone, decrease gastro-oesophageal reflux and enhance oesophageal clearing. As a result symptoms decrease, less antacid is needed and, if present, oesophagitis heals quicker. It has however certain side effects such as abdominal cramps and diarrhoea but they are not as a rule major problems and tend to be dose related.

Noxious effects of refluxant

Bile is probably as important if not more important than acid. Exogenous irritants such as acid fruit drinks and strong alcohol beverages should not be indulged in.

Acid causes damage only if in high concentrations. If this is suspected acid inhibitors such as the H$_2$RAs are the drugs of choice. Otherwise acid buffers are sufficient or mucosal protection can be offered in the form of alginic foams. There probably exists too great a pre-occupation with acid while the damaging effects of pepsin seem to be forgotten. This may well explain the inconsistent results obtained from the use of antacids or acid inhibitors.

Until recently surgery offered the best remedy against damage from the regurgitation of bile and bile salts. Medicine can now challenge this monopoly. Bile salts can be made somewhat innocuous by the use of such binders as cholestiramine, while the bile salt pool can be reduced by ursodeoxycholic acid.

Impaired defence mechanism

Finally, if mucosal defence mechanism is impaired medical therapy has an uphill struggle.

Anti-inflammatory drugs such as steroids and immunosuppressors, if taken, may have to be stopped.

Antibiotics can alter oesophageal flora and lead to invasion by candida. This should be checked and, if present, treated.

Mucus secretion may be improved by such drugs as Carbenoxolone or protected by foams.

A neglected area seems to be salivary secretion which may be a greater factor in oesophageal clearance than we realize. It ceases during sleep when the supine position accentuates regurgitation. Perhaps more attention should be paid to drugs increasing salivary flow.

So much so for the role of conservative treatment. But when impairment of sphincter tone and of the mucosal defence mechanism exists, can medical therapy offer anything better than the surgical restoration of competence permanently?

So far there has been no controlled comparison between modern medical treatment and modern surgical intervention chiefly because the latter is called upon when the former has failed. In the long run, to be totally successful, medical treatment must aim at increasing LOS tone; but it works only if that tone is very low to start with, a state of affairs which tends to require antireflux surgery. Apart from the effects of cholinergic drugs, of metoclopromide and of guaiacol, no increase in LOS tone has been recorded when other drugs are used, be they antacids, parietal cell blockers or mucosal protectors.

The results of medical treatment are difficult to compare and to assess and much confusion exists. Well-controlled trials are hard to come by and objective data are often lacking. Some authors hold that less than 5% of symptomatic cases fail to respond to medical treatment; yet 10–15% of all patients referred with oesophagitis have a peptic stricture, while 50% of these will not respond to the administration of the H$_2$RAs.

Why not surgery then, since it is more likely to offer complete if not lasting symptomatic relief?

Two aspects of surgery are more than just points of philosophy. In the patient with overlay the placebo effect of surgery cannot be assessed nor be judged; while in the patient requiring as competent an anti-reflux procedure as can be offered we may stop the symptoms of reflux at the price of imposing new symptoms that are unacceptable. Clearcut indications for surgery are thus necessary and demand that careful and purposeful medical management should be considered or should have failed. A combined medical/surgical unit, in the long run, offers the best assessment of the patient and in such a unit indications for surgery are found in the following order:

(a) Symptoms – chiefly those of regurgitation – not controlled.
(b) Intractable oesophagitis.
(c) Peptic ulcer or stricture.
(d) Histological changes.
(e) Unresponsive pulmonary symptoms.
(f) Anatomico-physiological factors.

Failure to control reflux symptoms are of two types:

(a) Those that do not become asymptomatic on active treatment over a 3-month period.
(b) Those that relapse whenever treatment is relaxed, such treatment having been imposed for a minimum of 3 months and, if necessary, up to six months.

Intractable oesophagitis carries the risk of ulceration, stricturing, bleeding and rarely perforation; and requires an urgent decision. It results from failure to decrease frequency, or duration, or the irritant nature of reflux episodes. Its assessment must be clinical, endoscopic and pathological (biopsy), and a decision should be reached if there is no improvement after two months of aggressive treatment.

Peptic ulcer and stricture should be treated to a conclusion. The combined refluxer, that is the patient who refluxes both in the erect and the supine position; the chronic refluxer; and the presence of an over-sensitive mucosa or of a highly irritant refluxed fluid, demand an unequivocal decision as to permanent treatment. Unless the patient is a very poor surgical risk due to reasons such as advanced old age, cardiac and renal conditions etc., strictures should not be subjected to endless repeated dilatation without correction of the cause of the uncontrolled reflux.

There is now increasing evidence that repeated injury to the mucosa leads either to columnar cell invasion (Barrett's oesophagus) or to atrophy ushering in dysplasia. Both are pre-malignant states and if medical treatment fails to reverse the histology, surgery should be seriously considered before the condition becomes irreversible.

All too frequently pulmonary symptoms fail to be attributed to reflux that otherwise does not affect the oesophagus. The damage is often done at night with the patient aspirating small quantities of gastroduodenal fluid giving rise to nocturnal asthma or to chronic morning cough. Bronchitic episodes are common and lung abscesses may complicate the picture. The problem is essentially a mechanical one and before major cardiopulmonary complications are experienced, specially in the aged, surgery should be offered.

Finally, there are clearcut anatomicophysiological features that make surgery unavoidable.

The combined refluxer has already been mentioned. To this, and often associated with it, must be added a group of patients with an LOS manometric pressure of less than 5 mm Hg, or with no abdominal oesophagus. Several variants exist. A short abdominal oesophagus with a normal LOS pressure will yield to a raised intra-*abdominal* pressure. In the reverse situation, that is a normal length of abdominal oesophagus but a poor LOS tone, a raised intra*gastric* pressure produces reflux; while the short abdominal oesophagus with an incompetent LOS falls foul of all situations and needs corrective surgery.

In all the above indications antireflux surgery is the operation of choice. However, it is not suitable in certain specific conditions, in which should be offered alternative procedures which will be discussed later. These conditions are:

(a) Air swallowing, mistaken for reflux.
(b) Motility disorders such as diffuse spasm or late achalasia; or those associated with poor peristalsis.
(c) Non-dilatable strictures.
(d) Iatrogenic reflux resulting from surgical destruction of the anatomy of the normal cardia.

If antireflux surgery is proposed, what surgery?

The early operations for reflux were based on the restoration of normal anatomy. They assumed that the hernia was responsible for the reflux, failing to realize that only a minority with a sliding hiatus hernia suffered from reflux peptic oesophagitis. The hernia was reduced via a thoracic approach and a variety of procedures were adopted to fix a portion of the oesophagus below the diaphragm. Restoration of normal anatomy was expected to lead to restoration of normal physiology. The results were far from gratifying and earnt surgery a bad reputation from which it has not yet recovered. Furthermore a fair incidence of intercostal neuralgia became an albatross that haunted the unwary thoracic surgical mariner.

As the crura loop superiorly below the diaphragm and slant across the upper abdominal cavity to seek their distal posterior attachment behind the cardia, the next argument favoured repair of the hernia via an abdominal exposure. This did not alter the failure rate of the operation.

The difficulty in understanding the problem was reflected in a series of questionable thoracic approaches yielding varying degrees of unrewarding results. Finally, the surgical world realized that hiatal herniorrhaphy was *not* the answer, and that success required the reinforcement of the LOS with preservation of its dynamic and adaptable function.

This found its solution in the use of the fundus to wrap the lower oesophagus with a 3–5 cm muscular belt that is sensitive to intragastric pressure and adds to the LOS a varying degree of intrafundic compression offering a competence as near to physiological requirements as can be surgically fashioned.

Priority of place now probably goes to the Nissen fundoplication which is a complete wrap; and in experienced hands, careful selection and the use of a 40F bougie at the time of the plication, very gratifying results are obtained in more than 90% of patients. The Belsey Mark IV technique uses a partial wrap, while the Hill posterior gastropexy enjoys popularity in many centres. The Collis gastroplasty, requiring a thoracic approach, is tending to be displaced by an acid-reducing operation with a Roux-en-Y biliary diversion.

The Nissen's fundoplication has the advantage of simplicity and of being an abdominal operation. It demands that the lower oesophagus be mobilizable, making it possible to restore a length of abdominal oesophagus of at least 3 cm, while the cuff of fundus around it heightens the intraoesophageal pressure. That pressure should be no less than 35 mm Hg to reduce symptoms absolutely; a pressure that experienced hands will sense at operation without needing cumbersome manometric machinery, helped by the use of an intraluminal 40F bougie to prevent undue compression. In the first post-operative week this pressure may be as high as twice this level due to swelling or to spasm, but reduces back to its permanent level in the second week.

Collis' operation is meant for the uncommon problem of the short oesophagus. The upper lesser curve is tubulized into a new intra-abdominal oesophagus and it is now current practice to fundoplicate it. It is however a major thoracic procedure and needs expert hands. Similar results – in the region of 70–75% satisfaction – are claimed for the Roux-en-Y bile diversion with an acid-reducing operation, and it is a comparatively straightforward abdominal operation. It consists of an antrectomy plus a 50 cm Roux-en-Y conversion. It is well tolerated and provided the jejunal loop is 50 cm or more, bile is totally diverted.

We have now moved into a surgical era of excellent results, very different from the poor ones achieved by the pioneers of herniorrhaphy, but we have benefitted from their less rewarding experience. I believe that when cessation of medical treatment leads to early relapses we can incline to these more successful forms of surgical treatment with much less trepidation. The present situation with regards to gastro-oesophageal reflux is very comparable to that found in the therapy of duodenal ulceration after the advent of the more selective types of vagotomy.

A helicopter view of the subject can now be obtained with fairly clear areas of therapy (Fig. 14.1).

The lower oesophagus is either mobilizable or immobilizable. In the latter situation a thoracic approach may be imperative. In a mobilizable lesion with no complications, fundoplication via an abdominal approach is the method of choice. The presence of a stricture demands the addition of dilatation to a full 18 mm before plication; and dilatation is now a very safe procedure.

When associated lesions such as peptic ulceration or cholecystitis are present, they are dealt with at the time of the abdominal antireflux procedure.

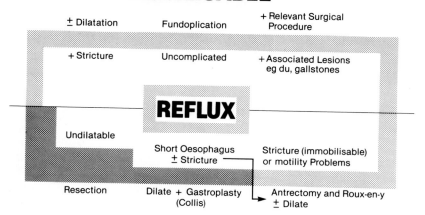

Fig. 14.1 A helicopter view of surgery for reflux problems.

When a stricture is dilatable but immobilizable, the simple procedure of antrectomy plus biliary diversion is far more preferable than a heroic transthoracic approach. Only when a stricture is neither dilatable nor mobilizable is resection required and is probably the only condition in which a thoracic approach is absolutely indicated.

Finally there remains the problem of lesions that should not be treated by antireflux surgery by virtue of the presence of motility disorders. Here, such type of surgery would change a disability into a catastrophe. This group of disorders is well suited to the diversion operations, though the success rate does not compare with those of the above procedures. Fortunately they are uncommon but are nonetheless taxing, and the failures are more than compensated for by the good results obtained in the treatment of other causes of gastro-oesophageal reflux.

REFERENCES

1. Winkelstein, A. (1935) Peptic esophagitis: a new clinical entity. *J. Am. Med. Assoc.*, **104**, 906.

PROBLEMS RELATING TO THE PERIPAPILLARY REGION

15

Papillary function and physiology

FRANK G. MOODY

The papilla of Vater and its sphincter of Oddi have engendered renewed interest during recent years as a consequence of advances in the ability to diagnose and treat presumed aberrations of their function [1]. Vater and Oddi would likely be pleased with these developments that involve structures that have become associated with their names. But therapies for papillary disease remain incomplete and for the most part empiric. Furthermore little is known about the normal physiology of the area. It is the purpose of this writing to review our current understanding of the function of the papilla of Vater as it may relate to hepatobiliary and pancreatic function, and the pathophysiology of disease.

ANATOMY OF THE PAPILLARY COMPLEX

The papilla of Vater in man presents as a small nipple-like protrusion from the mesenteric (pancreatic) border of the duodenum, usually at the junction of its middle and lower third. It can be recognized endoscopically or at operation through a duodenotomy by its small opening that is circumscribed cephalad by a crescent shaped mucosal fold. Ljunggren and his colleagues [2] have provided an elegant sequence of endoscopic photographs of the human papilla in their contribution to the 1976 Nice Symposium on this topic. The papillary mound is variable in size depending upon the bulk of smooth muscle within its sphincter (sphincter of Oddi) and the presence of disease. In the normal state, the papilla is rarely larger than a centimetre in size, while the minor papilla associated with the opening of the duct of Santorini is ordinarily only a few millimetres in diameter. The latter is most often a few centimetres cephalad and towards the left of the papilla of Vater.

There are a remarkable number of ways in which the bile and major pancreatic ducts enter the duodenum [3]. In many species, they form a confluence within the papilla of Vater beyond which there is an enlarged common channel, a true ampulla [4]. In man, the lumena of the bile and pancreatic ducts become narrower than their more proximal portion as they traverse the papilla, and the duct of Wirsung usually exits at or just within the inferior lip of the papilla, thereby precluding any possibility of a common channel or ampulla. Nonetheless, common usage has ascribed the name of ampulla of Vater to the inner aspect of the papilla of Vater of man, and the term ampullary sphincter is often used interchangeably to describe the sphincter of Oddi. In the following discussion, the term ampulla will not be used. The papilla will be considered as an anatomic unit that consists of the terminal end of the bile and pancreatic ducts, and the sphincter of Oddi.

Boyden has contributed greatly to our understanding of the intimate antomy of the papilla and its sphincter [5]. Fig. 15.1 reveals in elegant detail his reproduction of the relationships between these structures. Smooth muscle fibres envelop both the pancreatic and bile ducts, with the latter being predominant in man. There has been extensive discussion as to whether these fibres have their origin from the adjacent duodenal musculature or from the primitive mesoderm of the anlagen of the bile and pancreatic ducts [7, 8]. This may be an important question, since their site of origin may predispose how they respond to humoral or neural stimuli. Unfortunately, there is no way to distinguish these possibilities in man. As will be pointed out below, some species of mammal such as the opossum have a distinct biliary sphincter that responds in a manner different than adjacent duodenal muscle to pharamacological stimuli [9].

The transampullary septum, the thin veil of tissue that separates the terminal end of the bile duct from the duct of Wirsung, may be an important anatomic structure since it is shared by each as a common wall (Fig. 15.2) [10]. Possibly it acts as a baffle to prevent admixture or reflux of bile or pancreatic juice in the normal state. Clearly, the presence of a stone within the lower end of the bile duct could produce obstruction to the egress of pancreatic juice. In addition, the chronic passage of gallstones could lead to inflammation and fibrosis of the transampullary septum which also might interfere with pancreatic function. On the contrary, acute or chronic pancreatitis could lead to papillary abnormalities that might interfere with bile flow and liver function.

The papilla of Vater is lined by duodenal mucosa externally and the columnar epithelium of the bile and pancreatic ducts internally. While peripapillary neoplasms that arise within the duodenal or biliary epithelium are rare, neoplasms of pancreatic ductal origin in this region are all too common. There is speculation that a metabolite in bile might serve as an oncogenic agent for peripapillary pancreatic cancer. If this proves to be the case, then biliary–pancreatic reflux may assume an important, if not critical, role in the pathogenesis of this lethal disease.

In order for completeness, it is important to recognize that the papillary complex of man passes through the duodenal wall at an acute angle. The

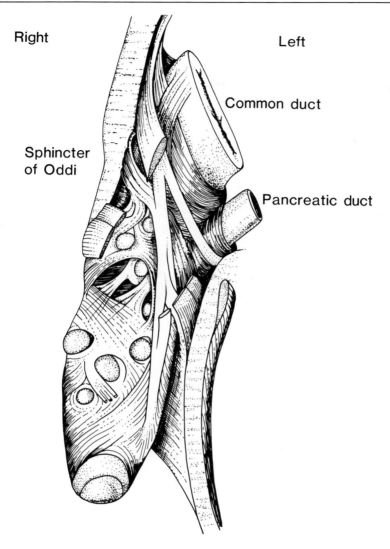

Right

Left

Common duct

Sphincter
of Oddi

Pancreatic duct

Fig. 15.1 Schematic of human papilla of Vater and its sphincter of Oddi represented in exquisite detail. Note that smooth muscle fibres envelop both the bile and pancreatic ducts. (Used with permission of *Surgery, Gynecology and Obstetrics*, [5], Fig. 17).

significance of this is not known. It is likely that the duodenal wall in this area contributes to the pressure gradient that exists within the papilla as described below. A contraction of the smooth muscle within the peripapillary area of the duodenum or a rise in intraduodenal pressure would therefore contribute to an increase in the transpapillary pressure and thereby prevent the reflux of duodenal contents that might occur during such an event [11].

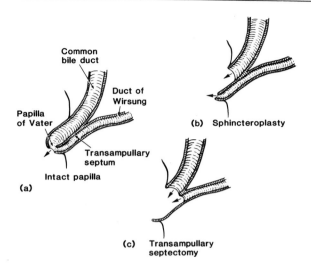

Fig. 15.2 Schematic of anatomical relationships within the papilla of Vater. Note the position of the transampullary septum forming the posterior wall of the bile duct and the anterior wall of the duct of Wirsung. (Used with permission of Lippencott/Harper and Row [8], Fig. 1).

FUNCTIONS OF THE SPHINCTER OF ODDI

The sphincter of Oddi represents a highly specialized mound of smooth muscle. Its length is variable, measuring from about 1–3 cm in autopsy studies. There is ample documentation that this is a true sphincter that can easily be distinguished morphologically from the adjacent muscle layers of the duodenal wall. It is not productive to distinguish components of sphincter function from that of the duodenal musculature in man since the sphincter is contained for the most part within it. This is not the case in lower orders of mammal such as the opossum where the biliary sphincter is external to the duodenal wall. During phylogeny, the biliary sphincter has gradually descended into the duodenal wall and has become a much less prominent structure (Fig. 15.3) [12]. This evolutionary development is understandable, since man being upright does not need a prominent biliary sphincter, while creatures that hang by their tails, such as the opossum, do.

The major role of the papilla of Vater and its sphincter of Oddi is to control the movement of bile, pancreatic juice and duodenal succus into and out of the bile ducts, gallbladder and pancreas. The anatomy of the papilla of Vater as described above is ideally suited to accomplish this task. A variety of neurohumoral interrelationships exist which coordinate the function of the sphincter of Oddi, and the demands placed upon it both at rest and during the digestion of a meal. A prominent feature of the transsphincteric area of the human papilla of Vater is a high pressure zone within both the bile and pancreatic ducts. A pressure profile of

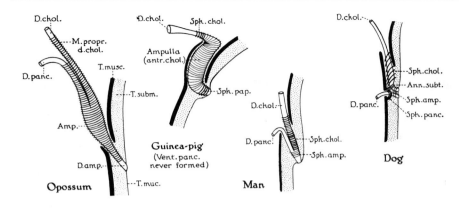

Fig. 15.3 Representation of the biliary sphincter in four species as portrayed by Boyden. Note that the biliary component of the sphincter gradually descends into the duodenal wall. (Used with permission of the C. V. Mosby Company, [10], Fig. 1).

the transpapillary portion of a human bile duct is shown in Fig. 15.4 [13]. The high pressure zone within the bile duct is several millimetres in length and is about 16 mm Hg, compared to intralumenal bile duct pressures of 12 mm Hg when duodenal pressures are zero. Clearly, these pressures offer a barrier to both the egress and ingress of fluids through the opening of the papilla. In the interdigestive state (resting), bile, which is continuously secreted by the liver, moves into the gallbladder as a consequence of this high resistance within the papilla. The transampullary septum acts as a flutter valve, preventing the movement of bile into the pancreatic duct under these conditions. During the resting state, the sphincter of Oddi is in tonic contraction, as evidenced by cyclical waves of extraordinary pressure occurring 2–4 times per minute (Fig. 15.5) [13]. In lower species of mammals, these pressure waves may represent a peristaltic action thereby providing for a transport of bile into the duodenal lumen with each contraction [14]. Whether this occurs in man is still open to question. Cineradiographic studies of the human papilla clearly demonstrate a pumping action with movement of contrast into the duodenum (Fig. 15.6). Unfortunately, most of these studies have been accomplished after the gallbladder has been removed and with the presence of a tube within the common bile duct [15, 16]. It is likely, however, that the cyclical contractions of the papilla play an important role in metering the rate of delivery of bile and pancreatic juice into the duodenum.

NEUROHUMORAL CONTROL OF SPHINCTER FUNCTION

The intimate mechanisms of sphincter of Oddi function are poorly understood. For example, it is not known whether the sphincter complex of man requires autonomic innervation for its proper function. Furthermore, the neural inter-

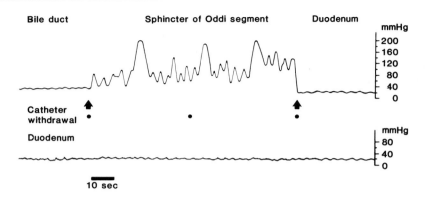

Fig. 15.4 Pull through pressure tracing of the sphincter of Oddi as obtained from a normal subject transendoscopically. (Used with permission of Elsevier North-Holland, Inc. [11], Fig. 2).

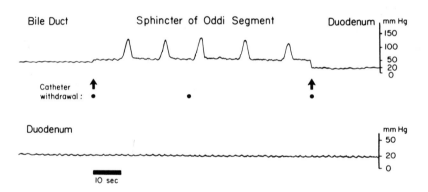

Fig. 15.5 High pressure cyclical waves within the sphincter of Oddi segment of a normal subject obtained by transpapillary cannulation through an endoscope. (Used with permission of Elsevier North-Holland, Inc., [11], Fig. 1).

relationships between cystic duct and papillary sphincter remains ambiguous. Apparently, the vagus plays a permissive and supplemental role to humoral stimuli that relax the sphincter; the sympathetic nerves may be an agonist to sphincter contraction in some species. Pitt and his colleagues have recently observed an increase in the amplitude of cyclical wave activity of the sphincter of Oddi of the prairie dog following truncal vagotomy (presented at the Fifteenth Meeting of the Association for Academic Surgery, November 1981). These results suggest that vagal tone was in some way inhibiting sphincter activity. It is possible, however, that truncal vagotomy was associated with an increase in gastrin release,

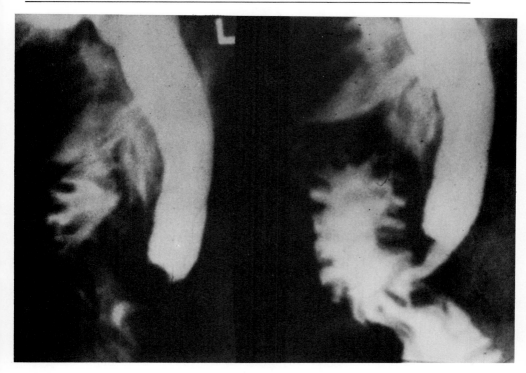

Fig. 15.6 Radiographic representation of the sphincter of Oddi. Rhythmic contractions of the sphincter can be observed during dynamic cinefluorography.

a hormone that acts as an agonist to the sphincter in this species. Tansy and Kendall have provided a recent review of the controversies in this area, of which there are many [17]. This is an obvious field for serious future research, since it is suspected that sphincter 'spasm' may be a stress-related event that can lead to abdominal pain.

Fortunately, much more is known about the effects of gastrointestinal hormones on sphincter function. This body of knowledge has been reviewed in an informative and elegant manner by Lin, a serious and productive student of the sphincter of Oddi [18]. The availability of pure hormones and peptides have provided a reasonable description of their effects on biliary motor function. Cholecystokinin has long been thought to be the primary hormone involved in biliary tract motility following the observation by Ivy and Oldberg that the intravenous injection of a crude extract of duodenum would induce gallbladder contraction [19]. Sandblom, Voegthin, and Ivy subsequently demonstrated the relaxing effect of cholecystokinin on the sphincter of Oddi of dog, thereby providing a scientific basis for the concept that the sphincter of Oddi relaxes to allow bile to flow into the duodenum as the gallbladder contracts [20]. It has also been shown that other related peptides such as gastrin and caerulein share this property of stimulating gallbladder contraction and sphincter relaxation. The octapeptide of cholecystokinin appears to be the most potent antagonist in this regard, while the response to pentagastrin is similar but less potent in each respect.

Not all investigators, however, have found cholecystokinin to be an antagonist to sphincter contraction. Watts and Dunphy observed an increased level of rhythmic contractions of the sphincter of Oddi when cholecystokinin was administered intravenously to dogs [21]. Touli and Watts subsequently were able to demonstrate that cholecystokinin induced a contraction of strips of common bile duct of man and dog studied *in vitro* [22]. Sarles and his colleagues have presented even stronger evidence that under some experimental circumstances caerulein, as well as cholecystokinin, can stimulate contractions of the sphincter of Oddi [23]. They studied the relationship between myoelectric activity, biliary pressures, and biliary flow in the anaesthetized rabbit in response to increasing doses of cholecystokinin and caerulein. A logarithmic incremental response was obtained in electrical activity and biliary pressure, with a comparable decrease in biliary flow.

My colleagues and I became fascinated by these diverse responses of the sphincter of Oddi to cholecystokinin and its related peptides. These observations reinforced the notion that indeed there could be an entity of biliary dyskinesia wherein the gallbladder and sphincter of Oddi could contract simultaneously. Duff repeated the experiments of Dubois and Hunt in which they had observed that the introduction of egg yolk and cream into the duodenum of the opossum would slow the rate of bile flow into the duodenum and cause an obvious increase in the contractile activity of the opossum's biliary sphincter. Duff made an important addition to his experimental design by measuring electrical as well as mechanical activity of the sphincter. His studies confirmed that intraduodenal instillation of egg yolk and cream led to a marked increase in the burst spike potentials emanating from the biliary sphincter of the opossum (unpublished results). This was associated with a decrease in flow through the papilla. Furthermore, transmission of spike potentials were antegrade, suggesting the presence of a pacemaker in the proximal muscular portion of the bile duct. A similar response was obtained to bolus doses of cholecystokinin. Becker subsequently performed dose response curves to cholecystokinin and its octapeptide, and to pentagastrin, and clearly demonstrated that each of these peptides were agonists for the biliary sphincter of the opossum [24]. Similar results have been obtained by Touli and his colleagues at the University of Wisconsin–Milwaukee [14].

Why should the biliary sphincter of the opossum and rabbit have this peculiar response to cholecystokinin? One possible explanation relates to the anatomy of the cystic duct which in each species lacks valves and serves as an open conduit into the common bile duct. The major resistance in the system is encountered at the terminal end of the bile duct. The biliary sphincter is therefore responsible for bile flow from the gallbladder as well as the biliary tree. In this scheme, cholecystokinin would prevent the sudden evacuation of bile from the gallbladder and the biliary tree as it increases both gallbladder and sphincter tone. Possibly the bolus dose techniques employed by those who have described the agonistic properties of cholecystokinin have unmasked a pharmacological property of the hormone that has little or no physiological significance. It is difficult, however, to rationalize in this way the increase in burst spike potentials and sphincter contractions that follow intraduodenal instillation of egg yolk and cream in the duodenum and presumed release of cholecystokinin.

Were the experiments of Watts and Dunphy [21] and Touli and Watts [22] a consequence of unique experimental design, or are there also circumstances during which the sphincter of Oddi of dog and man might contract in response to cholecystokinin? Ono, in fact, has demonstrated an increase in spike potentials from the papilla of Vater of man by placement of an extracellular electrode transendoscopically and injecting cholecystokinin intravenously [25]. I have attempted to confirm this observation by placing extracellular electrodes into the sphincter of Oddi within the papilla of Vater of patients undergoing sphinctero-plasty but have not been able to distinguish burst-spike potentials that are distinct from adjacent duodenal musculature. Bolus doses of 75 Ivy units of cholecysto-kinin have had no effect on the frequency of duodenal spike potentials under these conditions.

There is ample evidence to support the early observations of Sandblom, Voegthin, and Ivy that cholecystokinin is an antagonist to the papillary sphincter of the dog [20]. More recently, Geenen and his colleagues have provided direct evidence that the cyclical pressure wave forms observed at rest within the papilla of Vater cease after the intravenous administration of cholecystokinin (Fig. 15.7) [13]. They performed their experiments on awake subjects during the measure-ment of transpapillary pressures transendoscopically. Potts and I have made similar measurements at the time of operation upon the papilla, and while we can obtain transpapillary cyclical pressure tracings by passage of a 1.7 mm external diameter catheter through the papilla (Fig. 15.8), we have not been able to change the frequency or amplitude with a bolus dose of 75 Ivy units of cholecystokinin. These measurements were done with great difficulty, since frequent and vigorous rhythmic contractions of the duodenum followed the administration of cholecysto-kinin. These contractions induced extensive duodenal motion and periodic dislodgement of the sensing catheter from the high pressure zone within the papilla of Vater. We, therefore, can neither support or refute the observations of the Milwaukee group at this point in our studies. I believe that cholecystokinin is most likely an antagonist to the sphincter of Oddi in a physiological sense, although its primary action on the muscle of the sphincter when isolated from other factors may well be as an agonist. This concept would account for the numerous apparent discrepancies outlined above and would allow for a variety of responses, depending upon the microenvironment within which cholecystokinin finds itself at the time it approaches its target cell. Possibly the opossum and the rabbit have an inhibitory nerve that subverts the stimulus for contraction that should follow

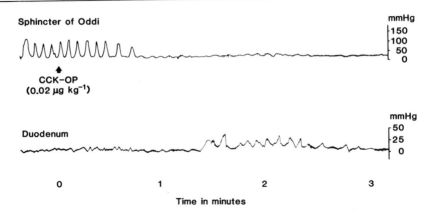

Fig. 15.7 Cholecystokinin inhibits the cyclical wave forms generated by the sphincter of Oddi of man. Simultaneous pressures were recorded by Geenen and his colleagues which revealed phasic contraction waves within the duodenum. (Used with permission of Elsevier North-Holland, Inc., [11], Fig. 4).

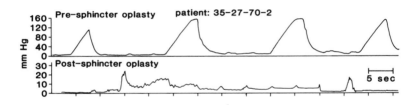

Fig. 15.8 Cyclical pressure waves recorded from the transsphincteric segment of the papilla of Vater of a patient undergoing transduodenal sphincteroplasty. The waves are abolished following sphincter division. These tracings were obtained by the passage of 1.7 mm OD Teflon catheter through the papilla of Vater from above. The catheter and perfusion technique was similar to that employed by Geenen and his colleagues [11].

cholecystokinin administration. Vagal, and alpha and beta sympathetic blockade have not provided useful information in this regard, since sphincter activity is not affected by agents that produce these states. Nor does autonomic blockade interfere with the sphincter response to exogenous or endogenous cholecystokinin. Touli and his colleagues have recently reported that total neural blockade with tetrodotoxin in the opossum reverses the usual antagonist response of the biliary sphincter to histamine, suggesting that in this species an as yet unidentified non-adrenergic, non-cholinergic neural pathway may be involved [26, 27].

I have attempted to be neither tedious nor exhaustive in my review of the physiology and pharmacology of the sphincter for, at this point in time, our knowledge of these areas is too fragmentary for critical review. It is clear from what is known that the study of human papillary function awaits further refinements in technology in order to establish its normal function and response to disease. The limitations of techniques for studying papillary function were also ignored in the above discussion in order to provide a cryptic overview of what is tentatively known in the area. Most of the methodology discussed above is designed to quantitate the resistance to flow through the papilla of Vater under varying experimental or clinical conditions. An increase in resistance, as evidenced by an increase in intrabiliary pressure or decrease in biliary flow, has been assumed to be related to a change in tonic activity of the sphincter of Oddi. Tansy and his colleagues have shown that an increase in blood flow to the papilla may change its lumenal resistance, possibly as a consequence of a narrowing of its lumen as the suffused tissues expand to fill it [28]. Edema associated with inflammation from a common duct stone or acute pancreatitis could also contribute to a remarkable increase in papillary resistance and an abnormal response to neurohumoral stimuli. Add to these imponderables the inherent errors of the methods used to measure intrabiliary pressure or flow in the intact human, and it is surprising that we have any knowledge of how the papilla functions in man.

INTRAOPERATIVE BILIARY MANOMETRY

Initially, evidence of papillary flow was ascertained by the 'Marriot bottle' technique in which pressure changes in the reservoir were monitored by the appearance of bubbles from a vent beneath its contained fluid. The oldest and most commonly employed techniques for measuring flow through the papilla of Vater were described by Caroli and his group in the early 1940s [29]. The principle is a simple one in which an isotonic solution is introduced into the common bile duct either during or after surgery at a constant pressure, and the rate of flow through the duct is measured. The addition of a radiocontrast agent to the perfusate offered a way to estimate the pressure at which fluid would first pass from the bile duct into the duodenum. This technique also allowed the opportunity to obtain radiographic visualization of the bile duct [30]. Utilization of this technique, with a variety of modifications, has shown that the resting pressure of the common duct of man is in the range of 10 mm Hg and the 'opening' pressure, or the pressure at which the sphincter allows flow into the duodenum, is about 15 mm Hg [31]. It is quite amazing that these numbers are quite reproducible between clinics and varying techniques which in most instances are performed following a celiotomy with the patient under anaesthesia [32]. The variations of the Caroli technique have recently been critically reviewed by McGlynn and his colleagues in a carefully controlled pig model, and they agree that each method provides a simple and reproducible way to qualitatively assess sphincter function in the normal [33]. Cushieri has been more critical in this regard and has recommended a continuous flow system that renders pressure an independent variable [34]. We have attempted to reproduce this approach with ambiguous results because it is difficult to know what perfusion rate would approach the normal. Furthermore, the technique does not allow an estimate of the level of intrabiliary pressure that will encourage flow into the duodenum.

I have found the following apparatus to be both simple and capable of providing a reproducible estimate of intrabiliary and flow pressures at the time of operation (Fig. 15.9). It consists of a sterile 30 ml syringe barrel which is held in an inverted position within a movable frame. The syringe tip is connected to a spinal manometer which is connected by a separate frame to the stand (an IV pole). Three-way stopcocks are used to interconnect the syringe, manometer, and intrabiliary catheter. A No. 5 infant feeding tube is usually placed into the bile duct through the cystic duct and directed into the lower bile duct so that its tip is about 3 cm from the papilla of Vater. The syringe barrel serves as a reservoir to which is added 30 ml of warm (37°C) saline. The manometer is positioned so that its zero point is at the level of the common duct. It is also convenient to have the zero of the syringe also at this level. Resting pressure is easily ascertained by filling the manometer to the 5 cm mark. When this column is opened to the intrabiliary catheter, the pressure usually rises to about 10 cm. If the manometer is then filled to 15 cm, the meniscus should drop slowly to 10 cm if a true resting pressure was obtained, and if there is no obstruction to flow within the lower bile duct or its papilla. If flow does not occur, then the manometer should be filled at 5 cm increments in order to determine which pressures encourage flow. Pressures in excess of 25–30 cm are abnormal and should encourage a careful review of the peroperative cholangiogram, which should always be obtained at the completion of the measurement of intrabiliary pressures.

TRANSENDOSCOPIC MANOMETRY

A variety of techniques have been described to measure transsphincteric pressures by the endoscopic route [13, 35, 36, 37]. The major advantages of this approach include its safety, the absence of a need for anaesthesia or a celiotomy, and the opportunity to make repetitive measurements before and after an intervention. The disadvantages relate to the need of passing an endoscope into the duodenum and a catheter through the orifices of the papilla. The general principle is quite different from intraoperative biliary manometry. The transendoscopic approach measures intrasphincteric wall pressure rather than the resistance of flow through the spincteric portion of the papilla of Vater. The best way to accomplish this is by the method described by Geenen and his colleagues [13]. They employ a 200 cm Teflon catheter whose external diameter is 1.6 mm, which is small enough to allow its passage through the side hole of a side viewing gastroscope. The tip of the catheter has graded markings at 1 mm intervals and a 1 mm side hole placed 3 mm from its tip which is sealed. The catheter is prefilled and slowly perfused at a rate of 0.25 ml min^{-1} by a pressurized delivery system developed by Arndorfer. The latter is designed to provide a high fidelity pressure tracing at infinitely slow flows.

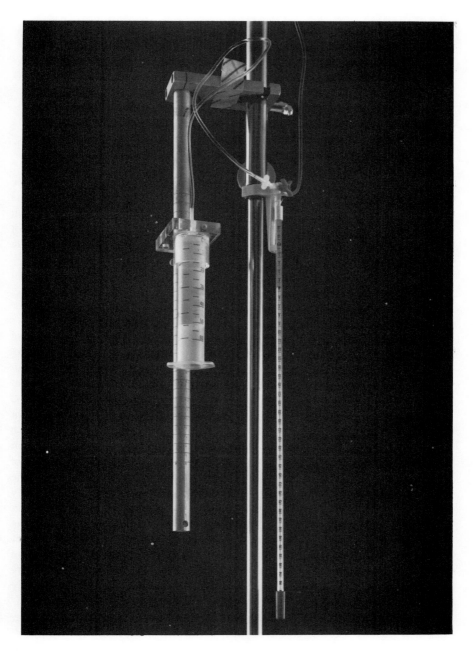

Fig. 15.9 This photograph reveals a simple apparatus for measuring intrabiliary pressure. The system consists of a 5 French feeding tube that is passed into the bile duct through the cystic duct. This is connected to a spinal manometer and a syringe barrel reservoir which is filled with sterile saline.

Pressures in the system are sensed and recorded on an appropriate polygraph. This technique provides six basic pieces of information:

(a) duodenal wall pressure
(b) transpapillary pressures within the bile and pancreatic ducts
(c) bile duct wall pressure
(d) pancreatic duct wall pressure
(e) length of the high pressure zones
(f) peak and trough pressures of the cyclical waves within the sphincteric zone of the papilla of Vater.

I am surprised that more endoscopists are not utilizing this technology, for the early reports from the Milwaukee group are indeed encouraging. Possibly the methodology is too complex for routine use. I imagine that the true explanation resides in scepticism as to whether diseases of the papilla actually exist that cannot be diagnosed by more conventional techniques such as endoscopic retrograde cholangiopancreatography.

DISEASES OF THE PAPILLA OF VATER AND ITS SPHINCTER

It is reasonable to assume that the papilla of Vater is at risk of developing most of the diseases which occur in other parts of the gastrointestinal tract. Furthermore, its strategic location at the terminus of the bile and pancreatic ducts provides a unique opportunity for it to be influenced by disease processes within either organ. A list of several abnormalities that affect the papilla are listed in Table 15.1. Peripapillary neoplastic diseases have been reasonably well described and will not be considered further in this discussion. Congenital abnormalities, on the contrary, are in an early phase of their description. One of the most common anomalies is failure of fusion of the ventral (duct of Wirsung) and dorsal (duct of Santorini) ducts, the so termed 'pancreatic divisum'. The papillary portion of the duct of Wirsung in this condition has a small, atretic lumen. Its opening usually allows the passage of only the smallest lacrimal probe which is about 1 mm in diameter. In three of the cases that I have operated upon, the ventral portion of the pancreas served by the duct of Wirsung was also diminished in substance. The duct of Santorini is usually enlarged and adequate in size for handling the flow of secretions from the body of the pancreas. It is likely that the pain suffered by patients with this anomaly is coming from the portion of the gland inadequately served by the duct of Wirsung.

The inflammatory lesions of the papilla are usually related to gallstone disease. Passage of a gallstone through the papilla can lead to inflammation in two ways, either by causing injury to its epithelium, or by inducing an episode of pancreatitis. The repair which follows an episode of inflammation from either cause may lead to fibrosis of the papilla, with secondary dilatation of the bile or pancreatic duct as a consequence of narrowing of their outlet. A third cause of stenosing papillitis is

Table 15.1 Abnormalities of the papilla of Vater

Congenital anomalies
Ectopic papilla
Pancreatic divisum
Neoplasms
Papilloma
Carcinoma
Inflammation
Cholesterolosis
Stenosing papillitis
Gallstones
Pancreatitis
Peptic ulcer
Motor dysfunction

cholesterolosis of the papilla of Vater. We are not as yet certain whether the submucosal cholesterol deposits which are evident on gross inspection and histological examination are secondary to injury from the passage of stones or are primary in nature. The lesion has been observed by me in three cases of cholesterolosis of the gallbladder in which no stones were found at the time of prior cholecystectomy, to suggest that the lesion could occur primarily within the papilla.

There still is uncertainty as to whether there are motor disturbances of the sphincter of Oddi that might contribute to biliary or pancreatic disease. Even the role of the common channel shared by the bile and pancreatic ducts has been challenged as a potential source of gallstone pancreatitis. It is now clear that the papilla of Vater in most people is not of sufficient size to house a gallstone which might allow the flow of bile under pressure into the pancreatic duct. The passage of a stone through the papilla probably induces pancreatitis in some way by obstructing the duct of Wirsung as it compresses the transampullary septum during transit.

Finally, we must deal with the issue of spasm of the sphincter of Oddi [38]. Is there such an entity? Can it contribute to recurrent episodes of chronic pain? These are questions for future study. Suffice to say that a large number of substances are known to cause an increase in the activity of the sphincter of Oddi [39]. Some examples include morphine, acetylcholine, intraduodenal hydrochloric acid, and even ethanol when instilled into the duodenum of the cat in high concentrations. As pointed out above, even cholecystokinin and its octapeptide and related peptides such as gastrin can induce increased motor activity within the biliary sphincter of the opossum and the rabbit. Electrical stimulation of the intra-abdominal vagi of a variety of species has been shown to induce contraction of the sphincter.

The stage is therefore set for a systematic and careful study of the role that the sphincter of Oddi might play in human disease. It is important, however, to approach these questions of papillary disease with caution and design well controlled studies to determine what underlying mechanisms are at play. This is especially true when chronic abdominal pain is the main or only symptom, unsupported by objective evidence of papillary dysfunction or pathology. Indiscriminate sphincterotomy, by either the transduodenal or endoscopic route, is doomed to failure if rigorous attempts are not carried out to uncover the pathophysiology of the presumed disease so treated.

REFERENCES

1. Moody, F. G. (1981) Surgical applications of sphincteroplasty and choledochoduoden-ostomy. *Surg. Clin. N. Am.*, **61**, (4), 909–22.
2. Ljunggren, B., Rey, J. F., Faure, X., Pangtay Tea, J. and Delmont, J. (1976) in *The Sphincter of Oddi*. (ed. J. Delmont), S. Karger, Basel-Munchen, Paris, London, New York, Sydney, pp. 363–42.
3. Hallenbeck, G. A. (1968) in *Handbook of Physiology*, Section 6, Vol. 2, Williams and Wilkins Co., Baltimore, pp. 1007–25.
4. Mann, F. C., Foster, J. P. and Brimhall, S. D. (1920) The relation of the common bile duct in common domestic and laboratory animals. *J. Lab. Clin. Med.*, **5**, 203–6.
5. Boyden, E. A. (1957) The anatomy of the choledochoduodenal junction in man. *Surg. Gynecol. Obstet.*, **104**, (6), 641–52.
6. Schwegler, R. A., Jr. and Boyden, E. A. (1937) The development of the pars intestinalis of the common bile duct in the human fetus, with special reference to the origin of the ampulla of Vater and the sphincter of Oddi. I. The involution of the ampulla. *Anat. Rec.*, **67**, 441–68.
7. Schwegler, R. A., Jr. and Boyden, E. A. (1937) The development of the pars intestinalis of the common bile duct in the human fetus, with special reference to the origin of the ampulla of Vater and the sphincter of Oddi. II. The early development of the musculus proprius. *Anat. Rec.*, **68**, 17–42.
8. Schwegler, R. A., Jr. and Boyden, E. A. (1937) The development of the pars intestinalis of the common bile duct in the human fetus, with special reference to the origin of the ampulla of Vater and the sphincter of Oddi. III. The composition of the musculus proprius. *Anat. Rec.*, **68**, 193–220.
9. Becker, J. M., Duff, W. M. and Moody, F. G. (1981) Myoelectric control of gastrointestinal and biliary motility: A review. *Surgery*, **89**, (4), 466–77.
10. Moody, F. G., Berenson, M. M. and McCloskey, D. (1977) Transampullary septectomy for postcholecystectomy pain. *Ann. Surg.*, **186**, (4), 415–23.
11. Lueth, H. C. (1932) Studies on the flow of bile into the duodenum and the existence of a sphincter of Oddi. *Am. J. Physiol.*, **99**, 237–52.
12. Boyden, E. A. (1937) The sphincter of Oddi in man and certain representative mammals. *Surgery*, **1**, 25–37.
13. Geenen, J. E., Hogan, W. J., Dodds, W. J., Stewart, E. T. and Arndorfer, R. C. (1980) Intraluminal pressure recording for the human sphincter of Oddi. *Gastroenterology*, **78**, 317–24.
14. Toouli, J., Honda, R., Dodds, W. J., Hogan, W. J. and Sarna, S. (1981) Spike-burst frequency of the opossum sphincter of Oddi in fasted and fed animals. *Gastroenterology*, **80**, 1305, (Abstract).
15. Beneventano, T. C., Jacobson, H. G., Hurwitt, E. S. and Schein, C. J. (1967) Cine-Cholangiomanometry: physiologic observations. *Am. J. Roentgenol.*, **100**, 673–9.

16. Burnett, W. and Shields, R. (1958) Movements of the common bile duct: studies with image intensifier. *Lancet*, **ii**, 387–90.
17. Tansy, M. F. and Kendall, F. M. (1975) in *Functions of Stomach and Intestine*. (ed. M. H. F. Friedman), Baltimore University Park Press, Baltimore, pp. 93–120.
18. Lin, T. M. (1975) Actions of gastrointestinal hormones and related peptides on the motor function of the biliary tract. *Gastroenterology*, **69**, 1006–22.
19. Ivy, A. C. and Oldberg, E. (1928) A hormone mechanism for gallbladder contraction and evacuation. *Am. J. Physiol.*, **86**, 599–613.
20. Sandblom, P., Voegthin, W. L. and Ivy, A. C. (1935) The effect of cholecystokinin on the choledochoduodenal mechanism (Oddi's sphincter). *Am. J. Physiol.*, **113**, 175–80.
21. Watts, J. M. and Dunphy, J. E. (1966) The role of the common bile duct in biliary dynamics. *Surg. Gynecol. Obstet.*, **122**, 1207–18.
22. Touli, J. and Watts, J. M. (1971) *In vitro* motility studies on canine and human extrahepatic tracts. *Aust. NZ J. Surg.*, **40**, 380–7.
23. Sarles, J. C., Bidart, J. M., Devaux, M. A., Eichinard, L. and Castagnini, A. (1976) Action of cholecystokinin and caerulein on the rabbit sphincter of Oddi. *Digestion*, **14**, 415–23.
24. Becker, J. M. and Moody, F. G. (1980) The dose/response effects of gastrointestinal hormones on the opossum biliary sphincter. *Curr. Surg.*, **37**, 60–3.
25. Ono, N. (1970) The discharge of bile into the duodenum and electrical activities of the muscle of Oddi and duodenum. *Jpn. J. Smooth. Muscle. Res.*, **6**, 123–8.
26. Behar, J. and Biancani, P. (1980) Effect of cholecystokinin and the octapeptide of cholecystokinin on the feline sphincter of Oddi and gallbladder. *J. Clin. Invest.*, **66**, 1231–9.
27. Toouli, J., Honda, R., Dodds, W. J., Hogan, W. J. *et al.* (1980) Action of histamine on phasic contractile activity in the opossum sphincter of Oddi. *Gastroenterology*, **78**, 1279, (Abstract).
28. Tansy, M. F., Salkin, L., Innes, D. L., Martin, J. S. *et al.* (1975) The mucosal lining of the intramural common bile duct as a determinant of ductal opening pressure. *Dig. Dis.*, **20**, (7), 613–25.
29. Caroli, J. (1946) La radiomanometrie biliare. *Sem. Hop. Paris*, **22**, 1985.
30. Mallet-Guy, P. (1952) Value of peroperative manometric and roentgenographic examination in the diagnosis of pathologic changes and functional disturbances of the biliary tract. *Surg. Gynecol. Obstet.*, **94**, 385–93.
31. White, T. T., Waisman, H., Hopton, D. and Kavlie, H. (1972) Radiomanometry, flow rates, and cholangiography in the evaluation of common bile duct disease. *Am. J. Surg.*, **123**, 73–9.
32. Schein, C. J. and Beneventano, T. C. (1970) Biliary manometry: its role in clinical surgery. *Surgery*, **67**, (2), 255–60.
33. McGlynn, M., Jefferies, S., Rose, M., and Ham, J. (1978) The experimental assessment of techniques of measuring biliary pressure. *Aust. NZ J. Surg.*, **48**, 581–5.
34. Cushieri, A., Hughes, J. H. and Cohen, M. (1972) Biliary-pressure studies during cholecystectomy. *Br. J. Surg.*, **59**, 267–73.
35. Nebel, O. T. (1975) Manometric evaluation of the papilla of Vater. *Gastroenterol. Endosc.*, **21**, 126–8.
36. Hagenmuller, F., Ossenburg, F. W. and Classen, M. (1977) Duodenoscopic manometry of the common bile duct in the sphincter of Oddi. *3rd Gastroenterologic Symposium*, Nice 1976. S. Karger, New York, pp. 72–6.
37. Carr-Locke, D. L. and Gregg, J. A. (1981) Endoscopic manometry of pancreatic and biliary sphincter zones in man: basal results in healthy volunteers. *Dig. Dis. Sci.*, **26**, (1), 7–15.

38. Dahl-Iverson, E., Sorenson, A. H. and Westengaard, E. (1958) Pressure measurement in the biliary tract in patients after cholecystolithotomy and in patients with dyskinesia. *Acta. Chir. Scand.*, **114**, 181–90.
39. Luoma, P. (1971) Studies on drugs affecting the choledochoduodenal junction in rabbits. *Acta Pharmacol. Toxicol.*, **29**, Suppl. 1, 1–55.

16

Papillary stenosis

J. P. SCHUPPISSER and P. TONDELLI

The papilla of Vater has become the meeting point of endoscopists and surgeons in their care of patients with biliary disorders. Although approached from different sides this small structure which controls secretions of bile and pancreatic juice is well known to both and some of its diseases, like the impacted stone or papillary carcinoma, are well accepted by them. The issue of benign papillary stenosis which Del Valle and Donovan in their original description in 1926 called 'papillitis stenosans' has remained controversial despite numerous discussions among surgeons and, by now, also endoscopists. While surgeons on the European continent appeared somewhat overzealous in their haste to diagnose and incise papillary stenosis, this disease was declared nonexistent and papillotomy considered an unnecessary if not criminal procedure on the sphincter of Oddi by most of their Anglosaxon colleagues. In the past few years unexpected help for the proponents was derived from the endoscopists who started to recognize papillary stenosis even more frequently than their continental surgical counterparts. In addition they created a somewhat competitive situation by solving this particular papillary problem in a surgical manner namely by endoscopic papillotomy.

FACTS IN FAVOUR OF PAPILLARY STENOSIS

In order to make clear what we consider to be papillary stenosis the term is herewith defined:

Benign disease of the papilla – sclerosis or adenomyomatosis – which impedes the passage of bile and pancreatic juice and which creates symptoms.

The pros for the existence of papillary stenosis could hardly be presented better than by the following case report. Our patient, a 50-year-old lady, underwent cholecystectomy without cholangiography or common duct exploration in 1964. Since 1970 she suffered from recurrent attacks of upper abdominal pain and jaundice secondary to cholangitis. In 1980 these attacks became more frequent and early this year she was admitted with an acute pancreatitis. Evaluation at this time included intravenous cholangiogram and ERCP and revealed a distended common bile duct without stones and a normal pancreatic duct. It was not possible to canulate the common bile duct by endoscopic retrograde cholangiopancreatography (ERCP) and, papillary stenosis being suspected, the patient was referred to us. Operative findings included a wide common bile duct without stones and in the pressure-controlled cholangiogram no flow of dye into the duodenum at a pressure of 14, 20 and 30 cm of water (Fig. 16.1). Transpapillary flow at a pressure of 30 cm of water was zero and after application of CCK 6 ml min^{-1} which is clearly less than the minimally expected 14 ml. After choledochotomy it was not possible to pass the smallest Fogarty catheter which measures 2 mm in diameter through the papilla, which we consider ultimate proof of an obstructed papilla. Therefore, transduodenal papilloplasty was performed by incising the papilla with the help of a transpapillary probe and approximating duodenal and choledochal mucosa with interrupted fine absorbable sutures (Fig. 16.2). Microscopic examination revealed marked chronic inflammation with sclerosis of the papilla. The patient has been asymptomatic for 12 months now.

This case – in our view – clearly demonstrates the existence of papillary stenosis. The existence of this disease is specially obvious in those patients with postcholecystectomy symptoms who do not have common duct stones or pancreatic pathology and who are cured by papillotomy. Before endoscopic papillotomy was possible these patients were reoperated. In an own series of 131 biliary reoperations in ten years we found papillary stenosis as sole pathology in 15 patients or 11% which is in accordance with the published 10–39% (Table 16.1) [1, 2, 3, 4, 5, 6, 7].

Formerly these patients had to be reoperated on but three recent publications by Seefeld, Viceconte and Seiffert document the efficacy of endoscopic papillotomy. Between 79 and 87% of a total of 876 corresponding patients were found to be cured of their postcholecystectomy symptoms approximately one year after endoscopic papillotomy (Table 16.2) [8, 9].

AETIOLOGY OF PAPILLARY STENOSIS

The aetiology of papillary stenosis is local scarring secondary to injury caused by passing stones or surgical manipulation or encroachment of inflammation of a

---

Fig. 16.1 Intraoperative pressure controlled cholangiograms. Papillary stenosis: no flow of contrast medium to the duodenum on the radiographs taken at a pressure of 14, 20 and 30 cm of water.

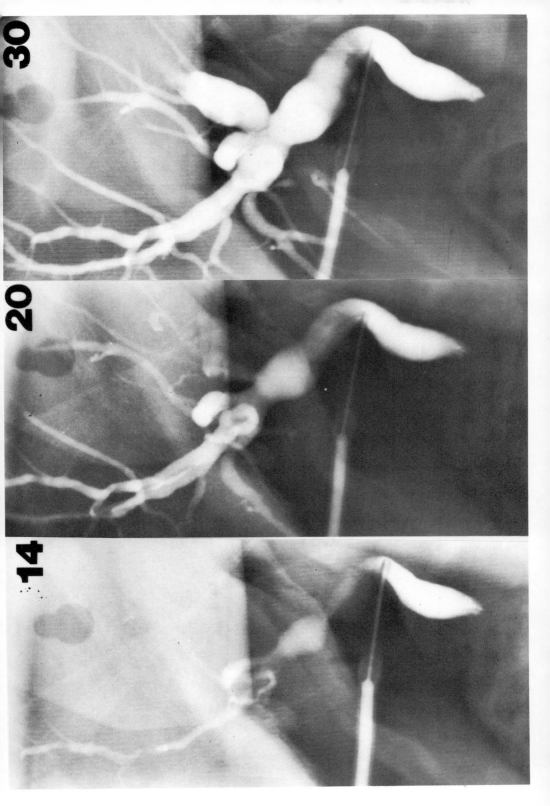

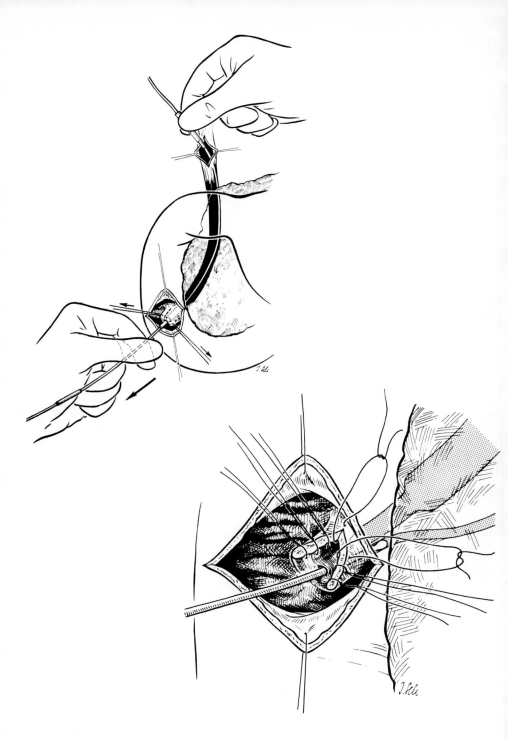

Fig. 16.2 Transduodenal papillotomy and papilloplasty. With the help of a transpapillary probe the papilla is exposed and incised (papillotomy). Choledochal and duodenal mucosa are then approximated with fine sutures after having identified the opening of pancreatic duct (papilloplasty). (Permission from Tondelli and Algöwer [10]).

Table 16.1 Frequency of papillary stenosis in biliary tract reoperations

Stefanini, P.	1974 [1]	14/36	39%
Alnor, P. C.	1974 [2]	74/201	37%
Grill, W.	1974 [3]	63/221	29%
Rückert, U.	1974 [4]	25/113	22%
Hess, W.	1977 [5]	37/310	12%
Tondelli, P.	1982 [6]	15/131	11%
Bordley, J.	1979 [7]	35/340	10%

Table 16.2 Results of endoscopic papillotomy in papillary stenosis

	Number of patients treated	Relief of symptoms in controlled patients	
Seefeld, U. 1981 [8]	14	11/14	79%
Viceconte, G. 1981 [9]	49	41/49	84%
Seiffert, E. 1981*	813	111/127	87%

* Personal communication.

neighbouring duodenal ulcer or an acute pancreatitis upon the papilla. Whether primary papillary stenosis exists remains controversial although histological findings like an adenomyomatosis would appear to be in favour of it. Primary and secondary papillary stenosis cannot be differentiated unequivocally because in the presence of biliary lithiasis it could conceivably have been the primary and thus causative factor and in the absence of biliary lithiasis a single small stone having passed the papilla can never be ruled out. Our experience with type and incidence of underlying pathology is shown in Table 16.3 [10].

DIAGNOSIS OF BENIGN PAPILLARY STENOSIS

If sympoms occur in a patient who has already had his gallbladder removed, the indication for another operative procedure will nowdays depend on the results of

Table 16.3 Underlying pathology in papillary stenosis – 97 cases operated 1968–1975 at the Department of Surgery, University Basel, Kantonsspital Basel, Basel, Switzerland

Gallstones present		
Gallbladder	51/97	53%
Gallbladder and common duct	38/97	39%
No gallstones		
Chronic pancreatitis	7/97	7%
No other pathology on biliary tract, pancreas	1/97	1%

an ERCP. Inability to canulate the papilla and delayed discharge of dye from the common duct are indicative of papillary stenosis. As evidenced by the rate of endoscopic papillotomies these criteria are quite subjective and tend to be interpreted on an individual basis.

Objective data could possibly be obtained by endoscopic manometry of the sphincter of Oddi which has not become a routine procedure due to its expense [11, 12]. Therefore it has not yet been possible to establish values of sphincteric pressures consistent with the diagnosis of papillary stenosis.

If on the other hand papillary stenosis exists in a patient with cholelithiasis, which occurs more frequently, symptoms are usually attributed to this latter condition. Therefore papillary stenosis has to be sought intraoperatively and the reported incidence of 0–40% is indicative for the lack of widely accepted diagnostic criteria [2, 10, 13, 14, 15, 16, 17, 18, 19].

The intraoperative examinations consist of:

(a) Cholangiography
(b) Flow measurement
(c) Probing of the papilla

If *cholangiography* is performed *manually* through a catheter in the cystic duct connected to a syringe judgement of papillary patency has to rely on the radiographic diameter. This type of evaluation is treacherous because with an anatomically measured diameter of 1–2 mm the papilla is normally very narrow and due to peristaltic changes it may appear occluded (Fig. 16.3). Therefore, the diameter of a normal papilla may easily simulate papillary stenosis on the cholangiogram. This is demonstrated by our following results: we reviewed the operative notes of patients with common duct exploration. In 148 records the surgeon noted a narrow, stenotic papilla on the intraoperative cholangiogram. This diagnosis was later, after opening the common duct and probing the papilla, shown to be wrong in 62 of 148, this is 42%. Probes with a diameter over 3 mm easily passed the papilla [10].

For many years *pressure controlled* cholangiography has been used at our surgical department in order to obtain objective information about the papilla. Radiographs are taken at pressures of 14, 20 and 30 cm of water. For this purpose we have built an easy-to-handle apparatus which is a modification of the one used by Caroli (Fig. 16.4). The main part is a vertically mobile syringe constructed according to the principles of a bottle of Mariotte, by which a constant pressure can be maintained despite falling fluid levels. Passage of dye into the duodenum is expected to occur at a pressure of 20 cm of water at the most and accordingly papillary stenosis is diagnosed if this is not observed (Fig. 16.1 and 16.5) [10]. Between 1968 and 1975 we diagnosed papillary stenosis in this manner in 4.9%, that is in 97 of 2106, biliary tract operations.

More recently we have relied more heavily on the observation of *flow* as diagnostic aid in papillary disorders. With the same apparatus we measure the

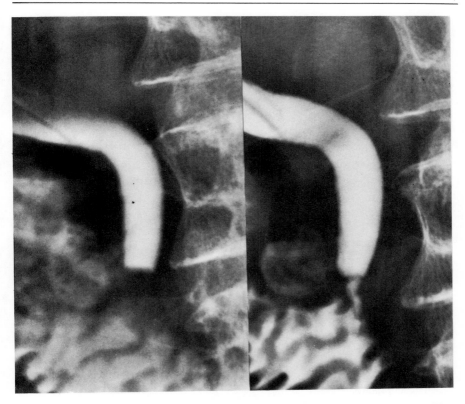

Fig. 16.3 Intraoperative cholangiogram. Papillary diameter may easily simulate papillary stenosis because the normal diameter is very narrow (1–2 mm in anatomical measurements) and because of papillary peristalsis.

quantity of dye flowing into the duodenum within one minute at a constant pressure of 30 cm H_2O which is defined as standard flow. The papillary diameter is proportional to the flow value and inversely proportional to the square root of the pressure used. In an experimental model with glass capillaries of different diameters we determined the corresponding flow e.g. 14 ml min^{-1} for a diameter of 0.5 mm. In a series of 161 simple cholecystectomies mean standard flow was 25 ± 10 ml min^{-1} corresponding with a functional papillary diameter of 0.6–0.7 mm. The normal value for standard flow was defined as greater than 14 ml min^{-1} respectively the normal value of the functional papillary diameter as greater than 0.5 mm [10].

Using these two measurements, i.e. pressure controlled cholangiography and standard flow, we have tested their accuracy in diagnosing papillary obstruction in a combined retrospective and prospective analysis of 193 (stone and stenosis) cases (Table 16.4). Papillary stenosis was proven by the inability to pass a probe

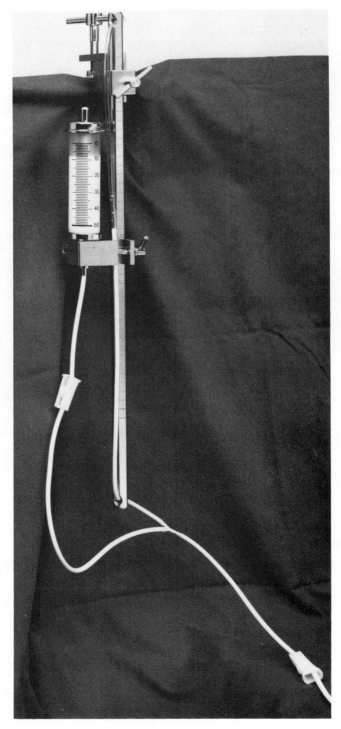

Fig. 16.4 Debitomanometer. Apparatus for intraoperative pressure controlled cholangiography and flow measurement (available from: Protek AG, Postfach 2016, CH-3001 Bern,
Switzerland).

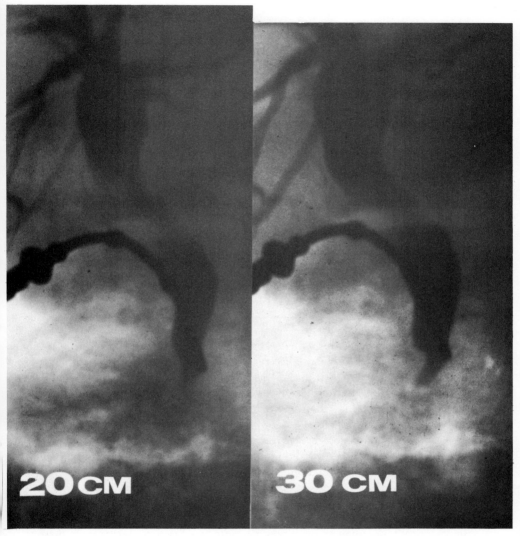

Fig. 16.5 Intraoperative pressure controlled cholangiograms. Papillary stenosis: no flow of contrast medium to the duodenum on the radiographs taken at a pressure of 20 and 30 cm of water.

with a diameter of 3 mm through the papilla. Histological confirmation was obtained in most of these cases. The accuracy of pressure controlled cholangiography alone was felt to be unsatisfactory with 80% and 85% in the prospective and retrospective parts of the study respectively and accordingly some small papillary stones and some of the papillary stenoses were missed. The addition of standard

Table 16.4 Accuracy of pressure controlled cholangiography and flow measurement in the intraoperative diagnosis of papillary obstruction (stone, stenosis), Department of Surgery, University Basel, Kantonsspital Basel, Basel, Switzerland

	n = 147 (retrospective study		n = 46 (prospective study)	
	False negative	Accuracy rate	False negative	Accuracy rate
Pressure controlled cholangiogram	22/147	85%	9/46	80%
Additional flow measurement	—	—	2/46	96%

Table 16.5 Flow before and after pharmacological test with CCK, Department of Surgery, University Basel, Kantonsspital Basel, Basel, Switzerland

Papilla	Number of patients	Flow in ml min^{-1} before CCK	after CCK
Normal	152	26 ± 9	30 ± 9
Functional obstruction (spasm)	40	9 ± 3	24 ± 6
Organic obstruction (stone, stenosis)	17	3 ± 3	4 ± 6

flow improved the diagnostic accuracy to 96%. In the prospective series seven additional papillary obstructions were found: four stones and three histologically confirmed stenoses [20].

One other important aspect of performing flow measurements concerns the possibility to differentiate between merely *functional spasms* and organic obstructions by the application of *CCK*. In a prospective study of 209 procedures on the biliary tree this pharmacological test was performed with the following results (Table 16.5): in 152 cases (73%) standard flow was normal, i.e. more than 14 ml min^{-1} at the initial examination. Application of CCK resulted in an insignificant increase from 26 to 30 ml min^{-1}. In 57 cases (27%) standard flow was initially subnormal but increased markedly in 40 cases after application of CCK, i.e. from 9–24 ml min^{-1} (Fig. 16.6). In the other 17 cases CCK did not influence standard flow i.e. 3 ml min^{-1} before and 4 ml min^{-1} after application. Accordingly these 17 cases underwent papillotomy and an organic obstruction was found in every single case: ten stones and seven stenoses [21]. This type of functional evaluation has resulted in a decreased rate of papillotomies from 4.6% of all biliary procedures between 1968 and 1975 to 2.5% in 1978 and 1979.

Fig. 16.6 Intraoperative pressure controlled cholangiograms. Papillary spasm: no flow of contrast medium to the duodenum on the radiograph taken at a pressure of 20 cm of water. Good flow after application of CCK 100 U iv.

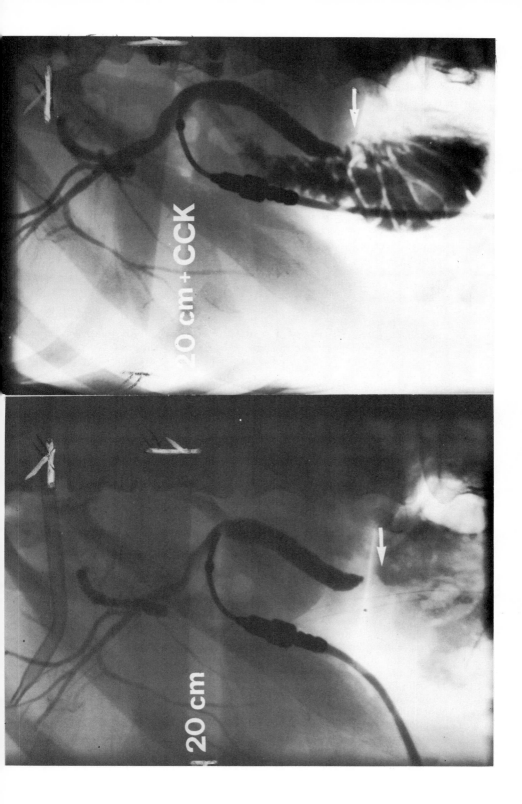

In summary we feel that, although rare, the papillary stenosis is a real entity. Not recognized at initial cholecystectomy it will later cause symptoms. Disparity in its reported incidence is due to lack of comparable objective diagnostic criteria. We consider flow measurements together with CCK the most reliable intraoperative evaluation of papillary function. Intraoperative probing of the papilla and matching microscopic findings serve as additional verification.

REFERENCES

1. Stefanini, P., Carboni, P., Petrassi, N., De Bernardinis, G. (1974) Transduodenal sphincteroplasty. Its use in the treatment of lithiasis and benign obstruction of the common duct. *Am. J. Surg.*, **128**, 672.
2. Alnor, P. C. (1972) Die papillitis stenosans Vateri. *Beiträge Klin. Chir.*, **219**, 229.
3. Grill, W. (1974) Reinterventionen an den gallenwegen. *Chirurg.*, **45**, 163.
4. Rückert, U. and Trede M. (1974) Zur reoperation an den gallenwegen. *Beiträge Klin. Chir.*, **221**, 281.
5. Hess, W. (1977) Nachoperation an der gallenwegen, *Praktische Chirurgie*, Heft 91, F. Enke, Stuttgart.
6. Tondelli, P., Gygli, Th., Harder, F. and Allgöwer M. (1983) Reoperationen an den gallenwegen: indikationen und resultate. *Helv. Chir. Acta*, (in press).
7. Bordley, J. and White T. T. (1979) Causes of 340 reoperations on the extrahepatic bile ducts. *Ann. Surg.*, **189**, 442.
8. Seefeld, U., Bühler, H., Woodtli, W. and Deyhle, P. (1981) Endoskopische papillotomie bei narbiger papillenstenose nach cholezystektomie. *Z. Gastroenterol.*, **19**, 505.
9. Viceconte, G., Viceconte, G. W., Pietropaolo, V. and Montori A. (1981) *Br. J. Surg.*, **68**, 376.
10. Tondelli, P. and Allgöwer, M. (1980) *Gallenwegschirurgie.* Springer-Verlag, Berlin, Heidelberg, New York.
11. Hagenmüller, F., Ossenberg, F. W. and Classen M. (1977) in *The Sphincter of Oddi* (ed. J. Delmont), Karger, Basel, New York.
12. Greenen, J., Hogan, W. J., Dodds, W. M., Stewart E. and Arndorfer, R. C. (1983) Intraluminal pressure recording from the human sphincter of oddi, (in press).
13. Kern, E. (1965) Operationstaktik der gallenwegsoperationen. *Langenbecks Arch. Chir.*, **313**, 264.
14. Spohn, K. and Müller-Kluge, M. (1965) Technik und ergebnisse bei 2000 operationen an den gallenwegen. *Langenbecks Arch. Chir.*, **313**, 300.
15. Hess, W. (1967) Probleme der operationswahl in der gallenchirurgie. *Chirurg*, **78**, 197.
16. Müller-Beissenhirtz, P., Berger, H. J. and Alnor, P. C. (1967) Das problem der papillotomie im rahmen der erkrankungen der ableitenden gallenwege. *Langenbecks Arch. Chir.*, **318**, 217.
17. Arianoff, A. (1968) *La Sphincterotomie de l'Oddi en Chirurgie Biliaire.* S. A. Arscia, Brussels.
18. Böhmig, H. J., Fritsch, A., Kux, M. and Stacher, G. (1969) Indikationen und ergebnisse der transduodenalen sphinkterotomie. *Langenbecks Arch. Chir.*, **323**, 173.
19. Cirenei, A. and Hess, W. (1977) Chirurgie du foie, des voies biliaires et du pancreas. Piccin Editore, Padova.
20. Tondelli, P., Schuppisser, J. P., Lüscher, N. and Allgöwer, M. (1979) Treffsicherheit peroperativer untersuchungen in der diagnose von gallengangssteinen und papillenobstruktionen. *Helv. Chir. Acta*, **46**, 795.
21. Schuppisser, J. P., Tondelli, P. and Allgöwer, M. (1981) Cholezystokinin in der intraoperativen prüfung der papillendurchgängigkeit. *Z. Gastroenterol.*, **9**, 504.

17

The papilla and the ventral pancreas

P. R. SALMON

Normal embryological development of the pancreas involves fusion of a dorsal and a ventral element of the pancreas during the second month of intrauterine life. The ventral rudiment rotates around the duodenum so that it comes to lie with its own duct (duct of Wirsung) alongside the dorsal rudiment with its ducts (duct of Santorini) (Fig. 17.1). Subsequent fusion of the dorsal and ventral duct system occurs near the tail of the ventral pancreas thus completing the adult anatomical pancreatic duct system. Failure of ductal union following rotation results in an

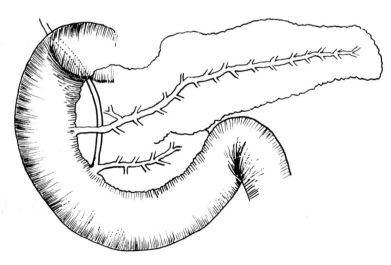

Fig. 17.1 Anatomy of the pancreatic ducts in IVP. The duct of Santorini drains through the minor papilla proximally in the duodenum, and the isolated ventral pancreas drains through the major papilla with the bile duct.

Table 17.1 Incidence of pancreas divisum at ERCP (after Cotton [5])

	Total	Isolated ventral pancreas
All ERCP	1215	47 (5.8%)
Primary biliary disease	291	6 (3.6%)
All recurrent pancreatitis	188	29 (16.4%)
Idiopathic recurrent pancreatitis	83	20 (25.6%)

Table 17.2 Incidence of isolated ventral pancreas (IVP) in published series

	Total	IVP (%)
Kasugai et al., 1972 [6]	92	Not mentioned
Oi, 1973 [7]	360	0.3
Phillip et al., 1974 [8]	813	2.7
Rosch et al., 1976 [3]	1850	3.4
Varley et al., 1976 [9]	102	2.9
Gregg, 1977 [4]	1100	3.0
Ohto et al., 1978 [10]	700	6.0
Rey et al., 1978 [11]	447	4.0
Cotton, 1980 [5]	810	5.8
Thompson et al., 1981 [12]	850	1.3

Table 17.3 Clinical details of 19 patients with IVP (after Cotton [5])

Age/Sex	Years of pain	Surgery	Abnormal PFT	Abnormal scans	Pancreatogram Ventral	Pancreatogram Dorsal
62 F	20	+	+		N	Abn
68 F	5	+			N	
72 F	2		+	US/CT	N	
22 M	5			CT	N	
68 M	4	+		US	N	Abn
50 M	3	+			N	
68 M	10		+		N	
34 M	1	+		US/CT	N	Abn
56 F	30	+		US/CT	N	Abn
57 F	5	+	+	US	N	Abn
50 F	1		+		N	
62 F	1				N	Abn
43 M	3	+	+	US	N	Abn
47 M	3	+				Abn
20 F	8	+			N	
40 F	5	+		US	N	Abn
43 M	4	+			N	
69 F	2					Abn
26 M	6	+		US		Abn

isolated ventral pancreas (IVP) which may be complete or partial, a condition first described by Charpy in 1898.

This anomaly has been found in 5.2–8% of cadavers [1, 2] and in 1.2–3.6% in other series [3–6]. Various groups [3] have suggested that drainage of the isolated dorsal pancreas (ventral part of head, body and tail) may become inadequate resulting in pancreatic pain and pancreatitis.

Whilst there is little hard evidence that this occurs except occasionally, there is growing circumstantial evidence that embryological pancreatic duct anomalies may be associated with symptomatic pancreatic disease.

INCIDENCE OF ISOLATED VENTRAL PANCREAS AT ERCP

Published figures should be related to the particular case selection relevant for that group. For this reason, the incidence of isolated ventral pancreas appears to be greater than it is for the general population. Cotton [5], for example, found an overall incidence of 5.8% in 810 pancreatograms (Table 17.1), whilst in those with 'idiopathic recurrent pancreatitis' where alcohol, gallstones and trauma were reasonably excluded, of 25.6%. Table 17.2 shows the incidence of isolated ventral pancreas in published series.

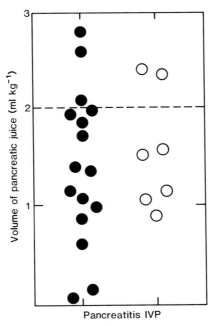

Fig. 17.2 Volume of duodenal juice in response to secretin, during standard secretin test. Patients with an IVP are compared with a group with chronic pancreatitis. The broken line marks the lower level of normal.

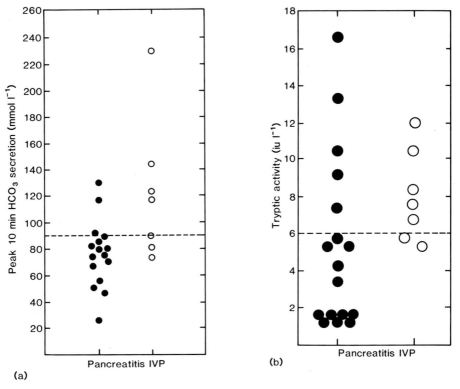

Fig. 17.3 (a) Peak 10 minute bicarbonate concentration in the duodenal juice in response to secretin during standard secretin test. Patients with an IVP are compared with a group with chronic pancreatitis. The broken line marks the lower level of normal. (b) Tryptic activity in the duodenal juice following a Lundh test meal. Patients with an IVP are compared with a group with chronic pancreatitis. The broken line marks the lower level of normal.

Evidence for an association between a clinical syndrome of pancreatic pain with or without demonstrable pancreatitis rests on epidemiological, anatomical and functional studies. Epidemiological evidence is scanty but nevertheless suggestive of a true association between IVP and a clinical syndrome. Table 17.3 shows a group of 19 patients with IVP in whom recurrent pancreatitis was identified by abnormalities of pancreatic function tests, pancreas scans or surgery. In a personal series [12] 11 cases of IVP were studied. In one case, laparotomy had demonstrated an abnormal pancreas prior to diagnosis of IVP whilst in a further two cases peroperative biopsy following diagnosis of IVP demonstrated chronic pancreatitis in the dorsal pancreas (body and tail).

There have been few functional studies performed in patients with IVP. Those that have been performed support in general the pattern related to pancreatic duct obstruction (Figs 17.2 and 17.3). For example, Thompson *et al.* [6] demonstrated a lower secretory volume with normal bicarbonate concentration during a secretin stimulation test of pancreatic function.

MANAGEMENT OF ISOLATED VENTRAL PANCREAS

Increased use of ERCP in recent years has provided the means of diagnosing IVP in patients with abdominal pain for which no non-pancreatic cause can be found. In those cases where pain is severe and recurrent surgical treatment can be considered, the options are either endoscopic or surgical sphincterotomy of the minor papilla, or surgical pancreatic drainage. At the present time, a limited distal pancreatectomy is probably the best initial procedure (preserving the spleen) in order to provide a good surgical biopsy of the pancreas and to allow pancreatography of the dorsal pancreas. If the duct system is dilated then pancreaticojejunostomy appears to be the most appropriate procedure. Pancreatic secretion should be reserved for patients with severe chronic pancreatitis.

Isolated ventral pancreas is probably an important clinical condition in a minority of patients with otherwise unexplained recurrent abdominal pain. Surgical intervention is probably justified in some of these patients where pain threatens the patient's job or where analgesic abuse results.

Further studies and observation are, however, necessary in order to provide long-term follow-up of these patients.

REFERENCES

1. Dawson, W. and Langman, J. (1961) An anatomical-radiological study on pancreatic duct pattern in man. *Anat. Rec.*, **139**, 59–68.
2. Millbourn, E. (1960) Calibre and appearances of the pancreatic ducts and relevant clinical problems. A roentgenographic and anatomical study. *Acta. Chir. Scand.*, **118**, 286–303.
3. Rosch, W., Koch, H., Shaffer, O. *et al.* (1976) The clinical significance of the pancreas divisum. *Gastrointest. Endosc.*, **22**, 206–7.
4. Gregg, J. A. (1977) Pancreas divisum: its association with pancreatitis. *Am. J. Surg.*, **134**, 539–43.
5. Cotton, P. B. (1980) Congenital anomaly of pancreas divisum as cause of obstructive pain and pancreatitis. *Gut*, **21**, 104–14.
6. Kasugai, T., Kuno, N., Kobayashi, S. and Hattori, K. (1972) Endoscopic pancreatocholangiography. I. The normal endoscopic pancreatocholangiogram. *Gastroenterology*, **63**, 217–26.
7. Oi, I. (1973) *Techniques of Endoscopic Pancreatocholangiography*. Igaku Shoin, Tokyo.
8. Phillip, J., Koch, H. and Classen, M. (1974) Variations and anomalies of the Papilla of Vater, the pancreas and the biliary duct system. *Endoscopy*, **6**, 70–7.
9. Varley, P. F., Rohrmann, C. A. Jr, Silvis, S. E. and Vennes, J. A. (1976) The normal endoscopic pancreatogram. *Radiology*, **118**, 295–300.

10. Ohto, M., Ono, T., Tsuchiya, Y. and Saisho, H. (1978) *Cholangiography and pancreatography*. Igaku Shoin, New York.
11. Rey, J. F., Blanch-Mouille, C., Garnier, C. and Delmont, J. (1978) Le pancreas divisum; realite anatomique et source de lesion pancreatique. *Ann. Gastroenterol. Hepatol.*, **14**, 196–7.
12. Thompson, M. H., Williamson, R. C. N. and Salmon, P. R. (1981) The clinical relevance of isolated ventral pancreas. *Br. J. Surg.*, **68**, 101–4.

18

Endoscopy and postcholecystectomy problems

R. F. McCLOY, V. JAFFE and L. H. BLUMGART

Patients undergoing cholecystectomy and choledocholithotomy for gallstones can be expected to be relieved of their symptoms in a majority of cases. However, 20% of all patients submitted to cholecystectomy have further symptoms and in 5% these are serious and persistent [1].

The range of problems that present in the patient after cholecystectomy are too varied to constitute a specific syndrome [2]. Postcholecystectomy problems represent any symptoms arising after cholecystectomy whether they are due to abnormality within the biliary tree or the result of an associated disease in commonly the pancreas, stomach or colon. It has been suggested that many of these patients have a psychosomatic origin for their symptoms [3]. If treatment of postcholecystectomy symptoms is to be successful, it is essential to try to ensure that they are related to demonstrable abnormalities. Reoperation after cholecystectomy is commonly hindered by adhesions, and abnormalities at the site of previously constructed surgical stomata are not easily recognized. Attempts at further operative cholangiography are difficult and diagnosis at laparotomy is often not made. This results in frustration to the surgeon and continued symptoms for the patient [4].

The major advances in imaging techniques during the last decade have brought new diagnostic approaches to the patient with postcholecystectomy problems. Once clinical history, physical examination and biochemical baselines have been established, we adopt an integrated approach to the radiological investigation of patients after cholecystectomy similar to that defined for the diagnosis of biliary tract obstruction [5, 6]. We no longer use intravenous cholangiography since it is usually valueless in the presence of jaundice and inaccurate and imprecise in many non-jaundiced patients [4]. Some patients are referred early after cholecystectomy with tubes or drains still in place. Repeat tubography may demonstrate a previously unrecognized abnormality within the biliary tree. More commonly, we use ultrasound to define the presence of dilated bile ducts and proceed to fine needle percutaneous transhepatic cholangiography (PTC) as the next investigation. In patients with postcholecystestomy problems, it is important to obtain not only cholangiography but pancreatography [7]. Thus, upper gastrointestinal endoscopy and ERCP are the investigations of choice in these patients and their use is not confined solely to those patients who do not have dilated ducts on ultrasonography [8]. Endoscopy and ERCP are carried out in the radiology department using standard techniques. During the examination, the stomach and duodenal cap are inspected for associated pathology, such as hiatus hernia, biliary gastritis and gastric or duodenal ulceration and it is important to inspect the papilla of Vater and surgically created stomata.

Patients referred to our department with postcholecystectomy problems have usually already undergone extensive investigation and multiple radiological studies. Previous radiographs including operative cholangiograms, T-tube and intravenous cholangiograms are studied and this may reveal an unsuspected diagnosis. Even if the biliary ductal system has been completely visualized and considered normal, ERCP is proceeded with provided there is clinical or biochemical evidence suggestive of upper gastrointestinal pathology, biliary obstruction or pancreatitis. We have currently analysed 57 cases referred to Hammersmith Hospital during an 18-month period (June 1979 to February 1981) as part of a total of 70 cases referred in a two-year period (June 1979 to July 1981). This extends our previously published experience of 52 cases [4] and 157 patients [9] with symptoms after cholecystectomy who were referred to the Glasgow Royal Infirmary.

The Hammersmith Hospital series (57 cases) represents an extremely complex group. There were 32 women and 25 men with a mean age of 52 years and an age range of 28–79 years. The delay in referral following initial cholecystectomy varied from immediately after the operation to 25 years later. Twenty-six out of the 57 cases (46%) had had another operation after cholecystectomy. The number of previous operations, including cholecystectomy, averaged 1.8 and the individual number of previous operations varied from one up to five.

The symptom complex in the postcholecystectomy patient usually comprises dyspepsia or biliary pain, although the more severe clamant presentation associated with jaundice, cholangitis or pancreatitis is not infrequent. Symptoms may appear immediately after cholecystectomy and this is especially likely if there has been iatrogenic damage to the biliary ductal system. Many patients, of course, have a combination of symptoms. However, if we look at the pattern of presentation in the one-third (16 cases) of our patients in whom the diagnosis was not obvious at the time of referral, three parameters were significant of pathology. In patients who had developed a new pain, distinct to that prior to cholecystectomy, eight out of ten were diagnosed as having definite pathology. If the pain was similar in nature to that before the first operation no organic pathology could be found in two out of five cases. Jaundice at the time of clinical examination on referral proved to be a sinister finding. Three patients had been jaundiced prior to cholecystectomy, remained jaundiced after the operation and were jaundiced at referral. Investigations revealed that all three patients had malignant tumours (one ampullary, two low cholangiocarcinomas). Routine serum biochemistry with estimation of bilirubin, alkaline phosphatase, aspartate transaminase (AST) and amylase was also a useful guide. In this difficult group of patients, five out of seven with one or more abnormal results, had definite pathology diagnosed.

The overall diagnosis in the Hammersmith series (57 cases) is shown in Table 18.1. Seventy per cent had either retained stones and or bile duct strictures and these patients are not considered further in this presentation. There was a variety of biliary and extrabiliary pathology and some patients also had more than one diagnosis. The complexity of this group is emphasized by the fact that only in two cases was no definitive diagnosis made. The incidence of periampullary problems and the value of endoscopic techniques are considered below.

Table 18.1 Postcholecystectomy problems – Hammersmith series

		Overall diagnosis in 57 cases
20	(35%)	Retained stones
20	(35%)	Bile duct strictures
		13 High
		3 Low
		4 Sphincteric
2	(3.5%)	Chronic pancreatitis
12	(21%)	Various
		5 Bile gastritis
		3 Tumours
		1 Extrabiliary fistula
		1 Liver atrophy
		1 Incisional hernia
2	(3.5%)	No definitive diagnosis
1	(2%)	Multiple pathology

Endoscopy and ERCP were performed in 23 of our patients (40%) and the findings are summarized in Table 18.2. Two patients had endoscopy alone. One had an obvious carcinoma of the ampulla of Vater and this was biopsied and no ERCP performed. The other was already known to have a retained stone in the common bile duct, diagnosed by an IVC prior to referral, and only duodenitis was seen endoscopically. Subsequent laparotomy in this latter patient demonstrated a biliary–enteric fistula between the common bile duct and duodenum which would have been diagnosed by ERCP had it been performed. In all patients an attempt is made to outline both the biliary and pancreatic ducts, although if a clear abnormality is demonstrated in either ductal system and the diagnosis is clear-cut, prolonged attempts to cannulate the remaining duct are not always pursued. In

Table 18.2 Hammersmith hospital series – 57 cases

---

2 Endoscopy

---

1 Duodenitis (IVC = retained stone)
1 Ca. ampulla

---

21 ERCP

---

  1 Failed
  4 (19%) Normal
12 (57%) Radiographic diagnosis
          5 (24%) Biliary–enteric fistulae
          5   Retained stones
          4   Chronic pancreatitis
          3   Biliary strictures
          1   Pseudocyst
  3 (14%) Endoscopic diagnosis – normal radiology
          2   Biliary gastritis
          1   Papillitis
          1   Choledochoduodenostomy

---

only one case did ERCP fail and in 19% both bile and pancreatic ducts were entirely normal. Fifty-seven percent had a radiographic diagnosis, but 14% had an endoscopic diagnosis in the presence of normal radiology. Biliary gastritis and papillitis were diagnoses based solely on endoscopic appearances. In this group of patients, one patient was deemed to have an inadequate choledochoduodenostomy stoma.

In the total Hammersmith series of 70 cases, there were 13 (19%) diagnosed as having periampullary problems – defined as pathology in the ampulla, the neighbouring duodenum, the head of pancreas or the retroduodenal and pancreatic portions of the common bile duct. All 13 cases had endoscopy/ERCP performed. The spectrum of these periampullary problems is detailed in Table 18.3. The main diagnosis was the pathology considered to be causing the patient's symptoms and the secondary pathology lists the associated findings. The three malignant tumours have already been discussed. The patient with a main diagnosis of papillitis had a surgical papillotomy performed and no other abnormality was found. The case with an inflamed papilla as secondary pathology had associated retained stones and pancreatitis. Clearly the most significant numbers of patients were those with scarring/stenosis of the papilla. These nine cases who had all undergone previous sphincter operations (one endoscopic and eight surgical papillotomies), all had periampullary problems and six biliary–enteric (choledochoduodenal) fistulae. Five of the nine papillotomies had become stenosed and one had endoscopic papillitis.

At the time of presentation, all six cases of biliary–enteric fistulae had pancreatitis; three also had cholangitis and two a previous history of jaundice.

Table 18.3 Hammersmith hospital series – 70 cases

13 Periampullary problems (19%)	
Main diagnosis	Secondary pathology
5 Scarred papillotomies	6 Choledochoduodenal fistulae
3 Tumours	5 Pancreatitis
1 Stenosed choledochoduodenostomy	1 Papillitis
1 Stenosed papilla	
1 Papillitis	
1 Pancreatitis	
1 Multiple pathology	

ERCP proved a successful technique for defining this pathology. The fistula tract and the papilla, with subsequent opacification of both bile and pancreatic ducts, were cannulated in all cases. We have now seen 13 biliary–enteric fistulae in our combined experience with 227 patients (Glasgow and Hammersmith) presenting with postcholecystecomy problems. In almost every case, the papilla and the Vaterian section of duct had been tampered with endoscopically or surgically, by deliberate sphincterotomy/sphincteroplasty, usually during transduodenal exploration of the common bile duct or instrumentation of the ampulla using rigid instruments at the time of supraduodenal exploration. Fig. 18.1 represents an artist's sketch of the endoscopic appearances seen in a patient with a normal ampulla of Vater and a choledochoduodenal fistula created in error, proximal to the true papilla. Fig. 18.2 is the ERCP obtained in this patient demonstrating the large false track (arrowed) of the fistula. The operative note stated that sphincteroplasty had been performed. We have seen no cases of primary papillary stenosis – all scarred or stenosed papillae had undergone an earlier operative insult.

We have previously suggested that nearly all endoscopic abnormalities of the papilla correlate with abnormalities at ERCP in every case [9]. Out of a total 108 examinations, ten were observed endoscopically to have a stenosed sphincteroplasty. Cannulation failed in three of these and an abnormality on ERCP – either a stone, fistula or chronic pancreatitis – was demonstrable in the remaining seven. In eight cases with red/inflamed/oedematous papillae, one case with an impacted stone could not be cannulated and the remaining seven had abnormalities on ERCP (as before). Four cases were considered to have 'protruberant' papillae. One with an impacted stone could not be cannulated and the remaining three all had abnormal ERCPs. Eight ampullae were thought small or stenosed with no previous operative procedure to the ampulla. One case could not be cannulated but the remaining seven all had pathology diagnosed (stone/fistula/pancreatitis). This experience has been supported by our present study.

Patients with postcholecystectomy problems present an intricate web of

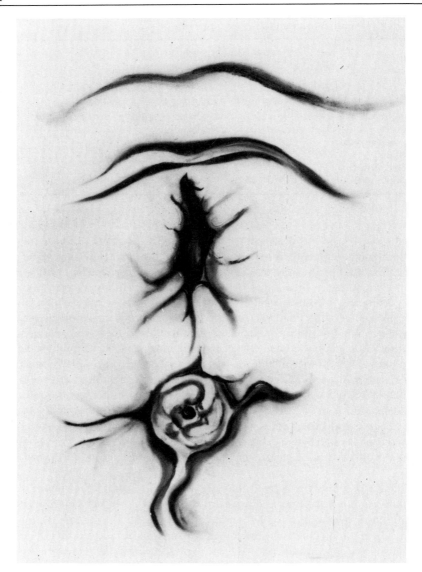

Fig. 18.1 An artist's sketch of the endoscopic appearances seen in a patient with a normal ampulla of Vater and a choledochoduodenal fistula created in error, proximal to the true papilla.

symptom and pathological complexes to be unwound by the investigator. However, selective investigation with ultrasound and PTC and particularly endoscopy and ERCP has provided a positive diagnosis of pathology in 97% of

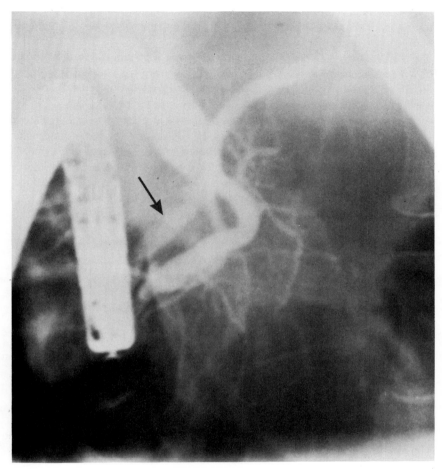

Fig. 18.2 The ERCP obtained demonstrates the large false track (arrowed) of the fistula.

patients with postcholecystectomy problems. In patients presenting with biliary colic or dyspepsia, especially when this is similar in nature to the symptoms before cholecystectomy, there is less frequently a demonstrable abnormality than in patients presenting with jaundice. In patients with cholangitis or pancreatitis, there was an abnormality on ERCP in every case. Coincidental upper gastrointestinal pathology is particularly likely in the dyspeptic group and duodenal ulcer not uncommon even in the presence of a previously normal barium meal. It is important in such patients that both the biliary tract and the pancreas are shown to be normal and not also involved [7, 10]. In our series, one patient in five had periampullary problems, nearly all of which were iatrogenic consequent upon previous surgery (or operative endoscopy).

The value of making a radiographic diagnosis in patients with postcholecystectomy problems is well recognized but the significance of endoscopic diagnoses remains less certain [9].

Finally, the management of a patient presenting with jaundice and cholangitis after cholecystectomy is clear. The question of how to treat a patient with 'old' pain who is diagnosed as having periampullary problems remains unanswered.

REFERENCES

1. Bodvall, B. (1973) The post-cholecystectomy syndrome. *Clin. Gastroenterol.*, **2**, 103–26.
2. Schofield, G. E. and Macleod R. G. (1966) Sequelae of cholecystectomy. *Br. J. Surg.*, **53**, 1042–5.
3. Valberg, L. S., Jabbari, M., Kerr, J. W., Curtis, A. C. *et al.* (1971) Biliary pain in young women in the absence of gall stones. *Gastroenterol.*, **60**, 1020–6.
4. Blumgart, L. H., Carachi, R., Imrie, C. W., Benjamin, I. S. and Duncan, J. G. (1977) Diagnosis and management of post-cholecystectomy symptoms: the place of endoscopy and retrograde choledochopancreatography. *Br. J. Surg.*, **64**, 809–16.
5. Benjamin, I. S., Allison, M. E. M., Moule, B. and Blumgart, L. H. (1978) The early use of fine needle percutaneous transhepatic cholangiography in an approach to the diagnosis of jaundice in a surgical unit. *Br. J. Surg.*, **65**, 92–8.
6. Benjamin, I. S. and Blumgart, L. H. (1978) in *Liver and Biliary Disease: A Pathophysiological Approach*. (eds R. Wright, G. Alberti, S. R. Karran and H. M. Sadler), WB Saunders Co. Ltd, London, p. 1219–46.
7. Ruddell, W. S. J., Ashton, M. G., Lintott, D. J. and Axon, A. T. R. (1980) Endoscopic retrograde cholangiography and pancreatography in investigation of post-cholecystectomy patients. *Lancet*, **i**, 444–7.
8. Blumgart, L. H. and McCloy, R. F. (1982) in *Surgery of the Gall Bladder and Bile Ducts*. (eds L. W. Way and J. E. Dunphy), W. B. Saunders, Philadelphia, (in press).
9. Hunt, D. R. and Blumgart, L. H. (1982) Endoscopic abnormalities in patients presenting with post-cholecystectomy problems. *Surg. Gastroenterol.*, **1**, 155–8.
10. Blumgart, L. H., Sokhi, G. S. and Duncan, J. G. (1976) Endoscopy and retrograde choledocho-pancreatography in the diagnosis of post-cholecystectomy symptoms. *Bull. Soc. Int. Chir.*, **34**, 587–91.

19

The papilla and malignancy: problems in clinical practice

C. W. VENABLES

The advent of duodenoscopy and ERCP has reawakened an interest in the diagnosis and management of pancreatic tumours. Of all the tumours arising in the pancreatic area, those occurring in the ampullary region are probably the most important ones. This is not because they are common (one series reporting only 34 out of 279 pancreatic tumours over a 20-year period [1]), but because they are more often amenable to resection and 'cure'.

However, these tumours are associated with a number of diagnostic and management problems.

SITE OF ORIGIN OF THE TUMOUR (Fig. 19.1)

By definition an ampullary tumour is one which first appears in the area of the ampulla of Vater but this does not mean that it has arisen from the sphincter itself, as there are a number of alternative sites. These are as follows.

Ampulla (62% [1])

These arise from the ampullary epithelium and are usually papilliferous in type. There is a rare benign papilloma but the majority are adenocarcinomatous in type, usually well differentiated on histological examination. Most of the tumours are small (17% have a 1 cm diameter [2]) when they first present and lymph node spread is present in some 28% [3].

Duodenum (15% [1])

Tumours can arise from the duodenal mucosa in the area of the ampulla. Macroscopically they can be impossible to differentiate from those arising from the

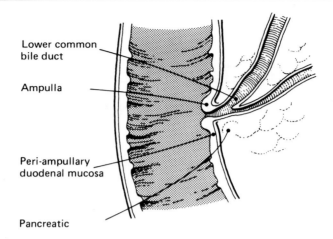

Lower common
bile duct

Ampulla

Peri-ampullary
duodenal mucosa

Pancreatic

Fig. 19.1 Sites from which tumours in the periampullary area may arise.

ampulla itself, but histologically they are obviously tumours of intestinal origin. Usually they have an ulcerated surface and they show lymph node spread in a similar proportion of tumours to those arising from the ampulla itself [3].

Lower common bile duct (24% [1])

As the bile duct emerges at the ampulla it is not surprising to find that some ampullary tumours arise from this site. Histologically they have a characteristic schirrhous appearance and lymph node metastases appear to be slightly less common (15% [3]).

Carcinoid tumours

Whilst these lesions are seldom reported in large series of ampullary tumours, we have had two out of 15 cases of tumours at this site. A review of reports on carcinoid tumours reveal that this is not an uncommon site for such lesions and that they appear to behave in a similar way to ileal carcinoid tumours with a similar risk of metastatic disease. They presumably arise from argentaffin Kultchitsky cells in the mucosal pits of the ampulla.

In both of our cases the tumours were less than 1 cm diameter and went deep within the ampulla without mucosal changes visible on the surface.

Pancreatic duct and acinar tumours

Tumours arising from the pancreatic duct and acinar tissue are normally excluded from the list of ampullary tumours. However, clinically it can be difficult to distinguish an acinar tumour arising from the head of the pancreas and infiltrating through the ampullary area from a primary tumour at this site.

The importance of distinguishing the site of origin (Fig. 19.2) and the histological type (Fig. 19.3) can be shown by the influences that these factors have upon overall survival.

DIAGNOSIS

The advent of fibreoptic duodenoscopy has revolutionized the diagnosis of ampullary tumours. Prior to the development of such equipment the diagnosis was usually made through less direct methods, such as the clinical features, changes on barium studies of the duodenal loop and the presence of occult blood in the stool. Most of these methods were unreliable with a diagnostic rate of only about 50% and many tumours were only found at the time of operation or at a 'second' operation in some cases!

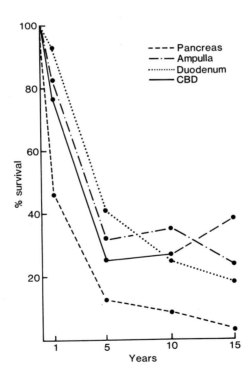

Fig. 19.2 Survival following radical resection of tumours in ampullary area according to site of origin (from [3] with permission).

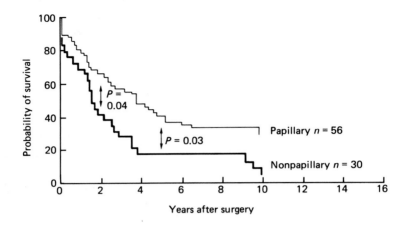

Fig. 19.3 Effect of histological type of ampullary tumour upon survival (from [2] with permission; © 1977, American Medical Association.

Nowadays there can be little excuse for not making the diagnosis prior to laparotomy! In my personal series of 15 cases the diagnosis was made with certainty at initial duodenoscopy in 80%. Three patients caused difficulty, two had carcinoid tumours which only produced gross distortion of the ampullary area without mucosal changes and the third had only an enlarged ampulla when first seen, although the diagnosis was made with certainty at a second duodenoscopy 12 months later!

Usually the presence of a tumour is obvious as the ampulla is enlarged and distorted and the mucosa has an increased papilliferous appearance or a typical ulcerated centre. In spite of the marked distortion and ulceration it is usually possible to cannulate the common bile duct through the tumour. A diagnosis can be confirmed by biopsy and brush cytology, the latter being particularly useful if the tumour lies within the ampulla.

Whilst the use of duodenoscopy and ERCP has rendered it impossible to make an accurate diagnosis in most patients, this is still not always made. Why is this?

Reliance on clinical features

Too often too much reliance is placed on a clinical diagnosis of the cause of obstructive jaundice. It is assumed that the patient has one of the more common causes; such as carcinoma of the head of the pancreas or gallstones, and laparotomy is undertaken without further investigation. Yet, as can be seen in Table 19.1, there are no distinct clinical features that can distinguish patients with such tumours from patients with these other conditions. Age is certainly no

Table 19.1 Clinical features seen in patients with tumours of the ampulla of Vater. A comparison of four different series.

	Akwari et al. [2]	Schlippert et al. [4]	Forrest and Longmire [1]	Personal series
No. cases	87	57	34	15
x̄ age (range)	60 years (31–86)	67 years (20–85)	61 years (33–82)	62 years (38–94)
Sex M/F	48/39	34/23	21/12	8/7
Jaundice	85%	91%	53%	80%
Pruritus	N.R.	51%	N.R.	53%
Pain	53%	65%	21%	27%
Weight loss	N.R.	94%	18%	93%
Gastrointestinal bleed	N.R.	9%	3%	7%

criteria, as patients have been described in all age groups beyond the second decade of life! Other features, such as weight loss, pain, pruritus, malaise, etc. are found in these other causes as well. In addition 10–15% of ampullary tumours may first present without clinical jaundice and the only clue may be a raised alkaline phosphatase or, slightly more commonly, a raised AST (SGOT) [2].

Coexistence of gallstones

Whilst most of these tumours occur in the absence of gallstones, they can occur in patients with stones or who have had a previous cholecystectomy. Two of my personal patients had undergone previous cholecystectomy and I have investigated another in whom the diagnosis was only made after removal of stones from the common bile duct for jaundice; when a postoperative T-tube cholangiogram showed no dye entering the duodenum! Similar cases have been reported in other collected series [4]. Thus the presence of gallstones cannot be used to exclude an ampullary tumour!

Errors in interpretation of investigations

A well recognized error is that of assuming that the jaundice is due to 'hepatitis' because of a raised aspartate transaminase (AST, SGOT). Akwari *et al.* noted that eight out of 40 patients with ampullary tumours had a greater than ten-fold rise in this enzyme on admission [2].

Nowadays a primary investigation of jaundice is that of ultrasound examination. This is a very useful investigation in distinguishing between 'intra-' and 'extra-' hepatic jaundice but requires careful interpretation if an ampullary tumour is not to be missed! In particular it is important that the ultrasonographer should try to determine how much of the extrahepatic bile duct system is dilated

Table 19.2 Complications of Whipple's resection (expressed as % of all complications)

Major complications	Nakase *et al.* [11] (n = 330)	Stephenson *et al.* [12] (n = 228)	Personal No ES	+ ES
Pancreatic or biliary leakage	39%	26%	21%	2 minor drain leaks
Haemorrhage	21%	15%	16%	0
Major sepsis	N.R.	13%	21%	0
Renal failure	5%	7%	5%	0
Cardio/respiratory	14%	13%	26%	0
Others	16%	— (Fatal)	11%	0

and what the relationship of this is to the duodenum. A confusing feature for him may be the marked pancreatic head enlargement that occurs with an ampullary tumour due to obstructive pancreatitis. Thus an enlarged pancreas on ultrasound should not put one off considering an ampullary tumour in the differential diagnosis!

The final investigation that may lead to confusion is the PTC. This investigation is becoming a fairly commonly used procedure in patients with extrahepatic jaundice. Like ultrasound, when carefully performed it can be very useful and, if it shows dilatation of the common bile duct right down to the ampullary area, then it should alert one to the diagnosis. However, if performed inexpertly then it is quite possible to be misled into thinking the obstruction to the common bile duct is much higher than it is. This is because the lower part of the duct may contain inspissated bile and mucus and the radiopaque dye may be delayed in diffusing into this area leading to the appearance of a high bile duct obstruction.

Missed at laparotomy

Even at operation the diagnosis can be missed! This can occur because the surgeon mistakes the enlarged head of the pancreas (due to obstructive pancreatitis from blockage of the pancreatic duct) for a tumour of the head of the pancreas. A very easy mistake to make! Or he may be unable to palpate an ampullary tumour through the duodenal wall. These tumours are usually small, ranging in size from only a few millimetres to up to 8 cm in diameter [4]. Many are less than 1 cm in diameter and through the duodenum they may be impossible to distinguish them from the normal nodular feel of the ampulla itself!

How then may these mistakes be avoided? One way would be to duodenoscope every patient with obstructive jaundice prior to a laparotomy. Whilst this is the most foolproof method, it is clearly not possible to do this in every centre and some selection is, therefore, inevitable. I believe that following a diagnostic 'flow chart' as in Fig. 19.4 and using duodenoscopy in this selected group of patients should reduce the risk of missing such tumours considerably. Those who do not have access to a duodenoscope should be able to see an abnormal ampulla if they have a modern narrow calibre wide-angle end-viewing endoscope. These instruments can usually be negotiated into the second part of the duodenum and should provide a tangential view of the ampullary area.

MANAGEMENT

There are two major problems in management. The first is how the patient should be made fit for operation and the second is what operation to do.

Preparation for operation

Over 90% of these patients are jaundiced at the time of their presentation [2, 3, 4, 5]. It has been clearly shown that jaundice increases the risks of operation and that there is a clear relationship between the levels of the serum bilirubin and the incidence of complications and mortality [6, 7].

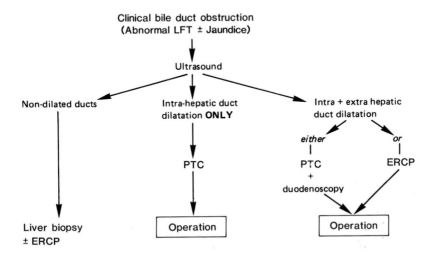

Fig. 19.4 A suggested 'flow chart' for the investigation of jaundice with the aim of avoiding missing an ampullary tumour before operation.

There are many complications that can occur but these fall into a number of subgroups (Table 19.2).

Anastomotic leakages and haemorrhagic complications can be partly attributed to the impaired protein synthesis that can occur in association with liver damage. Many of the infective complications probably arise from bacterial contamination occurring during surgery from colonization of the bile duct [8]. Finally, renal failure is a well recognized complication of surgery in the presence of jaundice due to the hepatorenal syndrome.

For these reasons it has been suggested that the jaundice should be corrected before resection is performed. There are several ways in which this may be achieved and each has its drawbacks (Table 19.3). In the past a surgical drainage procedure was performed as a first stage procedure. However, this has a number of major drawbacks which have reduced its popularity [7]. More recently transcutaneous bile drainage has been used instead. Whilst this may reduce the level of the jaundice it has its associated problems. These include difficulties in maintaining drainage for a sufficient period; increased risk of biliary infection and hepatic abscess formation and serious fluid and metabolic problems that may accompany this drainage, particularly if the bile is not returned to the gastrointestinal tract.

In our unit we have explored a third alternative, that of endoscopic sphincterotomy (ES) through the tumour [9]. In 1978 Ligoury and Loriga [10] reported successful ES in three patients with ampullary tumours and suggested that it might be valuable in preparation for operation. We have now attempted this procedure in a consecutive series of six patients and have been successful in all but one [11]. Our one failure was a carcinoid tumour of the ampulla when entry into the bile duct was impossible. To our pleasant surprise it has proved easier to perform than we had expected and, so far, bleeding has not proved to be the problem that might have been expected.

Table 19.3 Methods of bile drainage

Method	Problems
Surgical bypass (e.g. Cholecyst-enterostomy, choledocho-duodenostomy)	(a) Complications of surgery in jaundice (b) Delay in performing resection (c) Adhesions etc. at resection
External bile drainage (Percutaneous cannulation of ducts)	(a) Displacement of cannula (b) Infection of biliary tree (c) Metabolic problems (d) Difficult to maintain (e) Continued hospitalization
Endoscopic sphincterotomy	(a) May not be possible (b) Risk of bleeding (c) Possible risk of tumour dispersal?

The advantages of this approach are several. First it avoids any interference with subsequent abdominal surgery. Secondly, as the bile enters the intestine directly, there are no metabolic sequelae and there is an immediate improvement in fat absorption. Thirdly as the procedure is relatively 'minor' in nature the patient can rapidly return home whilst awaiting resolution of the jaundice. Finally it provides time during which a full discussion and planning of any subsequent resection can take place and is a palliative procedure should resection be contraindicated.

In our experience the jaundice fades rapidly and within six weeks the bilirubin has returned virtually to 'normal'. The improvement in the mental and physical health of these patients during this period has been most striking so that at the time of resection many regarded themselves as now 'fully fit'. This improvement is confirmed by the biochemical changes documented in this group (Fig. 19.5) when compared with an earlier series of 8 patients who underwent resection without ES.

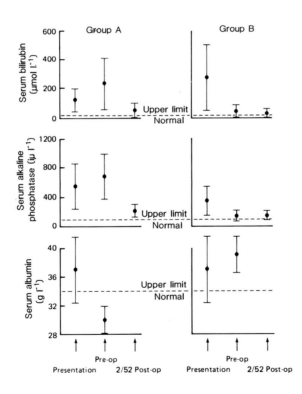

Fig. 19.5 Serial LFTs at presentation, immediately prior to resection and two weeks postoperatively in 8 patients who underwent resection without prior ES (Group A) and 5 who had a preliminary ES performed (Group B) (mean = ± 1 SD).

An additional, somewhat unexpected, finding was that in three of these patients the bile collected at surgery was now sterile, whilst in all those without previous ES the bile was heavily contaminated (Table 19.4).

What operation?

The choice lies between a 'palliative' or 'curative' procedure.

Palliative

These are mainly designed to relieve the jaundice. In the past these were entirely 'surgical' in nature and involved a laparotomy, but now ES is an alternative to this. Usually these procedures are reserved for the very old and infirm or for patients in whom widespread metastases have already occurred.

Curative

(a) *Local resection.* In many patients it is technically possible to remove an ampullary tumour through a transduodenal approach with reimplantation of both the pancreatic and common bile duct. However, such a resection does not remove any spread into the head of the pancreas or to local lymph nodes. For these reasons it is seldom used and when it has been [4] there is a high risk of local recurrence. It has been suggested that this procedure is only appropriate for patients in whom a pancreaticoduodenectomy cannot be justified.

(b) *Pancreaticoduodenectomy* (Whipple resection [11]). This is the only operative

Table 19.4 Bile culture results in Group A and Group B patients. All samples obtained at time of resection.

	Case no.	E.coli	Klebsiella	Str.faecalis	B.fragilis	Pseudomonas
				Organisms		
Group A	1			No specimen		
	2	√	√			
	3	√				
	4	√	√	√		
	5			No specimen		
	6	√				
	7	√	√		√	
	8					√
Group B	9			No growth		
	10		√	√		
	11			No growth		
	12			√		
	13			No growth		

procedure which can remove the whole tumour and its local lymphatic spread and therefore offers the best opportunity for a 'cure'. The majority of periampullary tumours (96% [4]) are suitable for such a resection.

The major problem is whether the risks of this major operative procedure are justified. A review of the literature reveals that the mortality associated with this operation can range as high as 30%, although in the larger series the average mortality is around 10–12% for ampullary tumours. In a large Japanese collected series [12] the overall mortality was 16% in 330 Whipple resections, although the authors had performed 12 such operations for ampullary tumours without any mortality; a similar finding to my own with no mortality in 15 cases!

Most deaths occur as a direct result of complications following surgery as can be seen in the study reported by Stephenson et al. [13]. The proportions of these various complications are similar to those reported in the large Japanese series [12] and in our own small series prior to ES when death has not occurred (Table 19.1). If the results we have seen in our patients following earlier ES can be produced by other centres, this procedure offers a real chance of significantly reducing the mortality associated with this operation.

The outcome following resection depends partly on the site of origin (Fig. 19.1) and partly upon the histological character of the tumour (Fig. 19.3) and the presence of lymph node metastases. Delayed surgical treatment and staged surgery have been associated with a lower overall survival in some series. However, there seems to be little doubt that the best results occur when the tumour is small and therefore earlier detection of these lesions by duodenoscopy should be associated with an improved prognosis.

REFERENCES

1. Forrest, J. F. and Longmire, W. P. (1979) Carcinoma of the pancreas and peri-ampullary region. *Ann. Surg.*, **189**, 129–38.
2. Akwari, O. E., Van Heerden, J. A., Adson, M. A. and Baggenstoss, A. H. (1977) Radical pancreato-duodenectomy for cancer of the papilla of Vater. *Arch. Surg.*, **112**, 451–6.
3. Warren, K. W., Dai Sun Choe, Plaza, J. and Relihan, M. (1974) Results of radical resection for peri-ampullary cancer. *Ann. Surg.*, **181**, 534–40.
4. Schlippert, W., Lucke, D., Anuras, S. and Christensen, J. (1978) Carcinoma of the papilla of Vater. A review of 57 cases. *Am. J. Surg.*, **135**, 763–70.
5. Stephenson, L. W., Blackstone, E. H. and Aldrete, J. A. (1977) Radical resection for peri-ampullary carcinoma: results in 53 patients. *Arch. Surg.*, **112**, 245–9.
6. Braasch, J. W. and Gray, B. N. (1977) Considerations that lower pancreatico-duodenectomy mortality. *Am. J. Surg.*, **133**, 480–5.
7. Aston, S. J. and Longmire, W. P. (1973) Pancreatico-duodenal resection. Twenty years' experience. *Arch. Surg.*, **106**, 813–17.
8. Keithley, M. R. (1977) Micro-organisms in the bile. *Ann. R. Coll. Surg. (Engl.)*, **59**, 328–34.
9. Alderson, D., Lavelle, M. I. and Venables, C. W. (1981) Endoscopic sphincterotomy before pancreoduodenectomy for ampullary carcinoma. *Br. Med. J.*, **282**, 1109–11.

10. Liguory, C. and Loriga, P. (1978) Endoscopic sphincterotomy: analysis of 155 cases. *Am. J. Surg.*, **136**, 609–13.
11. Whipple, A. D., Parsons, W. B. and Mullins, C. R. (1935) Treatment of carcinoma of the ampulla of Vater. *Ann. Surg.*, **102**, 763.
12. Nakase, A., Matsumoto, Y., Uchida, K. and Honjo, I. (1976) Surgical treatment of cancer of the pancreas and peri-ampullary region: cumulative results in 57 institutions in Japan. *Ann. Surg.*, **185**, 52–7.
13. Stephenson, L. W., Blackstone, E. H. and Aldrete, J. A. (1977) Radical resection for peri-ampullary carcinoma: results in 53 patients. *Arch. Surg.*, **112**, 245–9.

20

Endoscopic placement of biliary prostheses

K. HUIBREGTSE and G. N. J. TYTGAT

INTRODUCTION

The majority of patients presenting with malignant obstructive jaundice have unresectable tumours [1–4]. Palliative treatment of obstructive jaundice diminishes the complaints of itching and general malaise and so improves the quality of life. Palliative surgical bypass procedures carry a high operative morbidity and mortality and keep the patients hospitalized for a relatively long period of time, which can be better spent at home amongst their relatives [5]. Percutaneous transhepatic biliary drainage and insertion of biliary endoprostheses came as a first alternative to surgical bypass procedures. This technique, however, also carries appreciable hazards [6–8]. It was not surprising therefore, that with the more and more widespread use of ERCP, endoscopists also started looking for methods to drain malignant biliary obstructions. Endoscopic papillotomy was introduced to relieve jaundice in patients with obstructing tumours of the papilla of Vater. The next step was the introduction of nasobiliary drains for preoperative biliary drainage and for prevention of post-ERCP cholangitis. Since 1979 methods have also been developed to insert biliary endoprostheses via the transpapillary route [9–13]. The purpose of this communication is to describe the technique and the results of endoscopic insertion of large-bore biliary endoprostheses in 300 consecutive patients.

MATERIALS AND METHODS

Endoprosthesis

In general two types of endoprosthesis are used (Fig. 20.1): the pig tail endoprosthesis, the tail of which unfolds after insertion above the stenotic segment

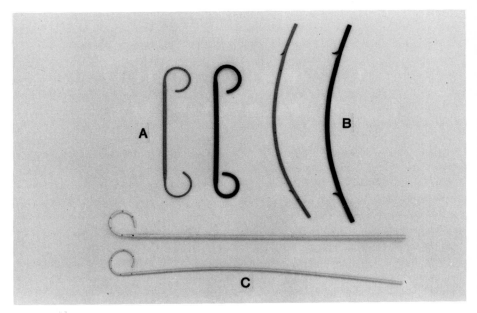

Fig. 20.1 Biliary endoprostheses. A: Double pigtail type. B: Straight Amsterdam type.C: Single pigtail type.

in the biliary tree to avoid dislodgement, and the straight Amsterdam type prosthesis with a side-flap in order to avoid dislodgement. Initial experience with these endoprostheses taught us that dislodgement of the endoprosthesis above the stenosis was still possible, and nowadays endoprostheses with two pig tails or two side-flaps, one at the proximal and one at the distal end, are preferentially used. Both types of endoprosthesis are available with diameters of 7 Fr and 10 Fr for use in duodenoscopes with respectively a 2.8 mm or 3.7 mm instrumentation channel.

Several materials are used for manufacturing the prostheses such as teflon, polyurethane, PVC and polyethylene. The straight Amsterdam type is made of polyethylene tubing.

Technique

Duodenoscopy and ERCP are performed for diagnostic purposes and to gather information about the biliary and pancreatic anatomy. A small papillotomy is carried out, which facilitates the introduction of the various catheters and which probably avoids the risk of pancreatitis due to occlusion of the pancreatic orifice by the endoprosthesis. A teflon catheter, with an atraumatic flexible guide-wire inside, is introduced into the common duct and manoeuvred through and above the biliary stenosis. In case of failure, first the guide-wire is manoeuvred through the stricture and then the catheter is advanced over the wire and pushed through the stricture. When using a pig tail type or a small calibre straight type endoprosthesis, the leading catheter has to be removed, leaving the guide-wire in the correct position. Then the endoprosthesis is pushed in position over the guide-wire. The guide-wire and the endoscope are removed, leaving the endoprosthesis *in situ*. The large-bore straight endoprosthesis is pushed into position over the stiff teflon catheter. This results in three main advantages. Firstly, the friction between the endoprosthesis and the teflon catheter is far less compared to the friction between a straightened pig tail endoprosthesis and the guide-wire. Secondly, the rather stiff catheter with the guide-wire inside assures a smooth bend between the duodenoscope and the papillotomy opening. This facilitates the introduction of the endoprosthesis into the common bile duct and decreases the risk of merely pushing the endoprosthesis and guiding device down into the distal duodenum. Thirdly, the combination of guide-wire, teflon catheter and endoprosthesis results in a rather stiff assembly. This allows the transfer of enough force to the tip of the endoprosthesis to pass even firm stenoses and makes dilatation of the stricture before introduction of the endoprosthesis superfluous in virtually all cases. A maximum of force can be generated by strong upward angulation of the tip of the endoscope while pulling the straightened endoscope. Complete sets of endoprosthesis, catheter, guide-wire and pusher tube are now commercially available for the pig tail endoprosthesis as the Soehendra set (Cook, Denmark) and for the straight endoprosthesis as the Huibregtse set (Surgimed, Denmark).

Indications

Only the indications in malignant obstructive jaundice will be discussed. Notwithstanding the progress in disinfection methods for endoscopes [14] and the awareness of performing ERCP procedures as sterile as possible, still cases of post-ERCP cholangitis in obstructed bile ducts occur. Only proper biliary drainage can further diminish this complication. We therefore prefer to introduce a large calibre endoprosthesis in the same session as the diagnostic ERCP in patients with malignant bile duct obstructions, unless surgery is already scheduled within 24 hours.

Further evaluation regarding fitness for surgery and resectability of the tumour can be performed, while the biliary tract is already decompressed. In patients unfit for surgery or with unresectable tumours we consider the endoprosthesis as the definitive palliative treatment modality.

PATIENTS AND RESULTS (Table 20.1)

Between August 1980 and December 1982 insertion of a large bore endoprosthesis was successful in 300 out of 336 patients (89%). Selective cannulation of the common duct and papillotomy was not possible in 21 patients.

Table 20.1

	Papillary tumour	Distal common duct	Mid common duct	Hilus
Male	9	80	25	28
Female	15	71	30	39
Age (yr)	71 (43–84)	69 (41–91)	71 (35–91)	66 (33–85)
Surgical bypass	2	13	2	0
30 day mortality	0	18 (11.9%)	12 (21.8%)	16 (23.8%)
Died (no.)	8	80	30	30
Median survival (days)	104	128	116	96
Range (days)	57–414	34–394	31–266	31–782
Alive (no.)	14	40	11	21
Median interval (days)	213	144	223	168
Range (days)	61–535	60–530	62–601	55–810
Early cholangitis	0	12 (7.9%)	8 (14.5%)	28 (41.8%)
Bilirubin decline	24 (100%)	143 (94.7%)	39 (71%)	48 (71.6%)
No bilirubin decline	0	8 (5.2%)	16 (29%)	19 (28.3%)

In five patients with a distal or mid common duct stricture and in 10 patients with a bifurcation stenosis, it was impossible to pass a guide-wire or catheter through such a stenosis. In 78 patients (26%) selective cannulation of the common duct was only successful after precut papillotomy.

Because of different technical difficulties and differences in tumour evolution, the patients are divided in four main subgroups regarding type of tumour and position of the stenosis. Three patients are lost for follow-up and are not included.

Papillary tumour (Fig. 20.2)

Twenty four patients (9 male, 15 female, mean age 71 years, range 43–84 years) with a papillary carcinoma were treated with a biliary endoprosthesis. In two of them a pancreatic endoprosthesis was also inserted in the highly dilated pancreatic duct. In 22 patients the endoprosthesis was the definitive treatment modality. Eight of them died after a median survival of 104 days (mean survival 160 days, range 57–414 days); 14 patients are still alive after a median time interval of 213 days (mean interval 254 days, range 61–535 days). Early complications did not occur. In all patients bilirubin levels normalized.

Distal common duct obstruction (Fig. 20.3)

In 151 patients (80 male, 71 female, mean age 69 years, range 41–91 years) an endoprosthesis was inserted through a distal malignant common duct stricture. All

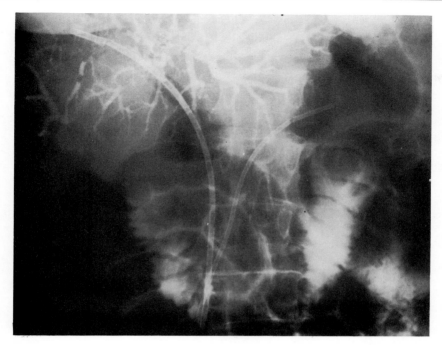

Fig. 20.2 A biliary and pancreatic endoprosthesis through a papillary carcinoma.

strictures were due to pancreatic cancer or primary common duct cancer. In 12 patients a pancreatic endoprosthesis was also introduced through the pancreatic duct stricture. In 13 patients a subsequent biliodigestive bypass was performed. Eighteen patients (11.9%) died in the first 30 days. In two patients death was due to a complication of the procedure. Eighty patients died after a median survival of 128 days (mean survival 146 days, range 34–394 days) and 40 patients were still alive after a median time interval of 144 days (mean interval 177 days, range 60–530 days). Early cholangitis developed in 12 (7.9%) patients. In one patient a severe bleeding and in another a perforation occurred. Both patients died. In 143 (94.7%) patients bilirubin levels declined. In eight (5.2%) patients the introduction of the endoprosthesis did not influence bilirubin levels.

Mid common duct stenosis (Fig. 20.4)

In 55 patients (25 male, 30 female, mean age 71 years, range 35–91 years) an endoprosthesis was introduced through a mid common duct stenosis. In 48 patients the stricture was due to a gallbladder or bile duct carcinoma, in seven patients it was due to an invading colon or gastric carcinoma or due to metastatic disease. In two patients a surgical bypass procedure was performed subsequently.

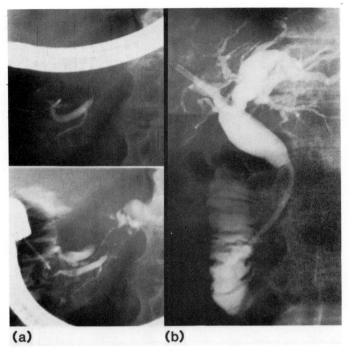

(a)   **(b)**

Fig. 20.3 (a) A double duct lesion due to a pancreatic carcinoma. (b) A well-functioning endoprosthesis bypasses the common bile duct obstruction.

The 30 day mortality was 21.8% (12 patients). One patient died due to a complication of the procedure. Thirty patients died after a median survival of 116 days (mean survival 111 days, range 31–266 days). Eleven patients were still alive after a median time interval of 223 days (mean time interval 277 days, range 62–601 days). Early cholangitis developed in eight (14.5%) patients. One of these patients died because of this complication. In 39 (70.9%) patients a bilirubin decline was seen. In 16 (29%) patients no bilirubin decline was seen after the procedure.

Bifurcation stenosis (Fig. 20.5)

In 67 patients (28 male, 39 female, mean age 66 years, range 33–85 years) a bifurcation stenosis was present. In 52 patients one endoprosthesis was inserted in one of the liver lobes. In 15 patients two endoprostheses were inserted to drain both liver lobes. In 51 patients the stenosis was due to a primary tumour, in 16 patients it was due to metastatic disease. No patient had a subsequent surgical bypass procedure. Sixteen patients (23.8%) died in the first month after introduction of the endoprosthesis. Three patients died due to the cholangitis, which developed after the procedure. Thirty patients died after a median survival of 96 days (mean

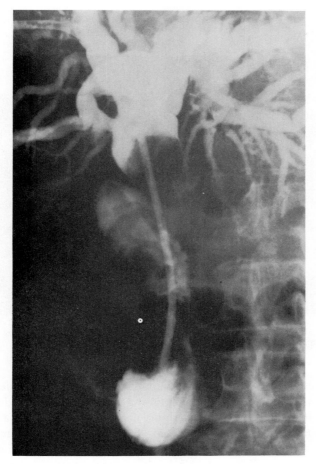

Fig. 20.4 A biliary endoprosthesis through a recurrent polypoid cholangiocarcinoma.

survival 143 days, range 31–782 days). Twenty-one patients were still alive after a median time interval of 168 days (mean interval 230 days, range 55–810 days). In 28 (41.8%) patients (27 of them with only one endoprosthesis) cholangitis developed after the introduction of the endoprosthesis. In 48 (72%) patients a bilirubin decline was seen. In 19 (28%) patients bilirubin levels remained unchanged.

EARLY COMPLICATIONS

Cholangitis

Routinely prophylactic antibiotics (gentamycine or tobramycine) were administered to the first 21 patients and to all patients with a bifurcation tumour and

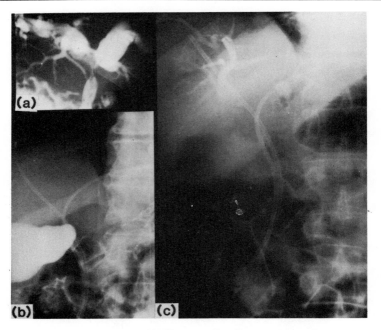

Fig. 20.5 (a) Bifurcation tumour. (b) Two small-calibre endoprostheses through this tumour. (c) Two large-calibre endoprostheses through this tumour.

only one endoprosthesis. Antibiotic administration was started immediately after the procedure. All ancillary equipment was gas-sterilized and the duodenoscope was disinfected in a home-made washing, disinfecting machine [14].

Nevertheless, cholangitis occurred in 48 (16%) patients. In most of these patients drainage of only a part of the biliary tree was obtained and cholangitis developed in the still occluded bile ducts. Four patients died because of untreatable cholangitis. In three patients with a bifurcation tumour and only one endoprosthesis, cholangitis could only be successfully treated after percutaneous drainage of the occluded lobe.

Endoprosthesis clogging

Early clogging of the endoprosthesis by blood clots occurred in two patients. In one patient the endoprosthesis was removed endoscopically. Attempts to pass the soft, necrotic, severely bleeding hepatoma were unsuccessful and the patient died with a septic cholangitis. The other patient also died due to sepsis. At post-mortem the endoprosthesis was found to be clogged by a blood clot.

Perforations

In one patient an endoprosthesis was introduced through a perforation opening, made during the insertion of a nasobiliary tube a few days before. This patient died after subsequent surgery, due to sepsis.

Papillotomy complications

For the introduction of a biliary endoprosthesis a small papillotomy is sufficient. Therefore complications of the papillotomy are rare. In three patients after a very difficult papillotomy, which was successful only after preceding precut, a complication occurred: one bleeding and two cases of acute pancreatitis. All three complications could be successfully treated medically.

LATE COMPLICATIONS

Endoprosthesis clogging

In 38 (12.6%) patients (29 patients once, five patients twice and four patients respectively 3, 4, 5 and 6 times) clogging of the endoprosthesis was shown endoscopically or by HIDA biliary scintiscanning. The median interval between introduction and clogging of the endoprosthesis was 121 days (mean interval 134 days, range 17–402 days). In 35 patients the endoprosthesis could easily be exchanged. In three patients exchange of the clogged endoprosthesis was impossible because of duodenal obstruction by the tumour. No clogging was seen in 47 (15.6%) patients, who survived more than six months. Of these 47 patients 20 patients died without recurrent jaundice after a median time interval of 272 days (mean interval 277 days, range 187–414 days). Twenty-seven patients are still alive without recurrent jaundice after a median time interval of 279 days (mean interval 305 days, range 182–601 days).

Endoprosthesis dislodgement

In two patients an endoprosthesis with only one side-flap moved above the stenosis. In one patient an endoprosthesis dislodged towards the duodenum and was evacuated spontaneously without the patient noticing it.

Acute cholecystitis

In one patient acute cholecystitis developed six months after insertion of the endoprosthesis because of cystic duct occlusion. Cholecystectomy was performed, but the patient died because of postoperative complications.

Duodenal stenosis

In six (4.3%) patients with a distal common duct obstruction a duodenal stenosis developed after a mean time interval of 207 days (range 116–298 days). In all six patients a gastroenterostomy could be performed. In four (16.6%) patients with a papillary carcinoma a duodenal obstruction occurred after a mean time interval of 324 days (range 86–402 days). In two patients a gastroenterostomy was performed. The other two patients were not operated on because of their very poor clinical condition.

Other late complications

In two patients with a pancreatic carcinoma, recurrent jaundice and cholangitis was due to the development of bifurcation lymph node secondaries. In one patient a longer endoprosthesis was inserted bypassing both stenoses, with a good clinical response. In the other patient it was impossible to insert an endoprosthesis through both strictures.

Biliary or duodenal injury by the endoprosthesis

In one patient during an endoscopic exchange of a clogged endoprosthesis, an ulcer was seen at the opposite site of the papilla. This ulcer was not clinically manifest and healed in two weeks. Clinically no further instances of duodenal injury were encountered.

In two patients at autopsy the endoprosthesis was found to have perforated the tumorous common duct wall. Clinically these perforations were not manifest.

DISCUSSION

In the great majority of the patients presenting with malignant jaundice only palliative treatment is possible. Evaluation by ultrasonography, cytological puncture, computer tomography and arteriography was performed in all our patients in good clinical condition. In only 24 patients (13.7%) with a distal common duct stenosis or papillary tumour, were the findings promising regarding the resectability of the tumour. However, at laparotomy the tumour proved to be unresectable in 19 patients. In five patients a curative pancreaticoduodenectomy was performed. At present only one of these five is alive and without recurrent disease. The low survival time of our patients (4.3 months) and the low resectability percentage (0.6%) must be due to patient selection. In fact, many patients were referred for endoscopic treatment because of their poor clinical condition.

Surgical bypass procedures carry a mortality percentage of up to 28%. Furthermore, at least two weeks additional hospitalization are necessary. Percutaneous transhepatic insertion of biliary endoprostheses is successful in about 75% of the cases, but carries a complication rate of 5–10% and a mortality rate of 2–3% [6, 7]. These figures in the literature are obtained by very experienced radiologists. In case of failure of this method, mortality and morbidity are much higher.

Endoscopic insertion of a biliary endoprosthesis was successful in 89% of the patients. Procedure-related death in our series was 2%. Complication rate in the patients with a distal common duct obstruction was 6.8%. One of the main advantages is that, in case of failure, no harm is done to the patient and the patient can be treated surgically or percutaneously without additional risks.

The endoscopic technique for insertion of biliary endoprostheses is now, in general, settled. Only minor improvements can be made regarding type of guide-wire, catheter or endoprosthesis. For an endoscopist with experience in performing ERCP and endoscopic papillotomy the procedure takes no longer than 30–45 minutes. The main cause of failure is the impossibility to cannulate the common duct and to perform a papillotomy. Selective cannulation of the common duct is more difficult in patients with malignant obstructive jaundice than in patients with gallstone disease. This can be due to displacement of the duodenum and gastric antrum or common bile duct by the tumour or by distal obstruction of the common bile duct. Furthermore, the absence of bile flow through the papilla seems to make cannulation more difficult. The second most important cause of failure is the impossibility to insert one or two endoprostheses through bifurcation tumours. Selective introduction of the guide-wire into the right and left hepatic duct is difficult, time-consuming and frequently unsuccessful. Guide-wires with a long or short flexible tip must be tried out and in most cases it is pure luck if both ducts can be drained. Even after selective introduction of the guide-wire, it can be difficult to push the catheter and endoprosthesis over the guide-wire. The long distance from the tip of the duodenoscope to the stricture, the curves in the common duct and the acute angle to the left or the right hepatic duct prohibits the conductance of sufficient force to the tip of the catheter to dilate the stenosis. Dilatation in these difficult cases was sometimes possible with home-made stiff teflon catheters of increasing diameter with a tapering metal tip. In these cases co-operation between the radiologist and the endoscopist can be fruitful. The radiologist can introduce a guide-wire through the stenosis and the endoscopist can then use this guide-wire for cannulation and introduction of the endoprosthesis.

The main late complication of biliary endoprostheses is the clogging pheno-menon. Clinically clogging results in recurrence of cholestasis and nearly always in cholangitis with fever and chills. The exact incidence of clogging was difficult to assess; this was partly because no investigations as to the cause of recurrent jaundice were made in patients in the terminal stage of the disease. Also, most patients died at home and autopsy was not performed.

In 38 (12.6%) patients clogging was proven after removal of the endoprosthesis or by HIDA scintiscanning after a median time interval of 121 days. On the other hand, in 47 (15.6%) patients the endoprosthesis functioned well for more than six months without recurrent jaundice. At present the ideal management for avoidance of the complications of the clogged endoprosthesis is close observation of the patients with frequent HIDA scintiscanning to detect impending clogging. Earlier exchange of the endoprosthesis should then prevent the occurrence of cholangitis. Routine exchange of the endoprosthesis every three months seems impracticable and unnecessary for many patients. To solve the problem of clogging, further research must be done as to the relation between bile composition, bile flow, liver function and the clogging of the endoprosthesis. In two patients with liver cirrhosis and a malignancy the endoprosthesis clogged every 4–6 weeks, suggesting that impaired liver function and bile flow play an important role in the clogging phenomenon. Furthermore, trials must be performed to find out the effect of other tubing materials, choleretic drugs, antibiotics or gallstone-dissolving agents.

The optimal internal diameter of the endoprosthesis probably lies between 2 and 3 mm. In our experience the 7 Fr endoprosthesis does not assure sufficient bile flow, and early cholangitis was a severe and not easily treatable complication. Also clogging of 7 Fr endoprosthesis was found to occur after a shorter time interval. The 10 Fr straight endoprosthesis seems to function well, probably because 2.4 mm diameter holes are present at both ends together with many side holes, to assure sufficient drainage. In two patients, in whom frequent clogging of the endoprosthesis occurred, the introduction of two or three large-bore endoprostheses did not avoid the clogging problem, suggesting that further increase in diameter of the endoprosthesis will not be of benefit in avoiding the clogging phenomenon.

In conclusion, the endoscopic biliary large-bore endoprosthesis is a major advance in the treatment of patients with malignant obstructive jaundice. Because of its low mortality and morbidity, in our opinion it is the method of choice for palliative treatment of mid and distal common duct strictures. At present the combination of percutaneous and endoscopic insertion of endoprostheses seems the best possible palliative treatment modality for bifurcation tumours.

REFERENCES

1. Feduska, N. J., Dent, T. L. and Lindenauer, S. M. (1971) Results of palliative operations for carcinoma of the pancreas. *Arch. Surg.*, **103**, 330–4.
2. Gudjonsson, B. (1981) Pancreatic carcinoma: diagnostic and therapeutic approach – A word of caution. *J. Clin. Gastroenterol.*, **3**, 301–5.
3. Williamson, B. W., Blumgart, L. H. and McKellar, N. J. (1980) Management of tumours of the liver. Combined use of arteriography and venography in the assessment of resectability especially in hilar tumours. *Am. J. Surg.*, **139**, 210–15.
4. Hermann, R. E. and Vogt, D. P. (1983) Cancer of the pancreas. *Comprehensive Therapy*, **9**, 66–74.
5. Sarr, M. G. and Cameron, J. L. (1982) Surgical management of unresectable carcinoma of the pancreas. *Surgery*, **91**, 123–33.
6. Ferrucci, J. T. and Mueller, P. R. (1981) Interventional radiology of the biliary tract. *Gastroenterology*, **82**, 974–85.
7. Mueller, P. R., van Sonnenberg, E. and Ferrucci, J. T. (1982) Percutaneous biliary drainage: Technical and catheter related problems in 200 procedures. *Am. J. Rad.*, **138**, 17–23.

8. Burcharth, F., Efsen, F., Christiansen, L. A. *et al.* (1981) Nonsurgical internal biliary drainage by endoprosthesis. *Surg. Gynecol. Obstet.*, **153**, 857–60.
9. Soehendra, N. and Reynders-Frederix, V. (1980) Palliative bile duct drainage – A new endoscopic method of introducing a transpapillary drain. *Endoscopy*, **12**, 8–11.
10. Huibregtse, K., Haverkamp, H. J. and Tytgat, G. N. (1981) Transpapillary positioning of a large 3.2 mm biliary endoprosthesis. *Endoscopy*, **13**, 217–19.
11. Huibregtse, K. and Tytgat, G. N. (1982) Palliative treatment of obstructive jaundice by transpapillary introduction of large bore bile duct endoprosthesis. *Gut*, **23**, 371–5.
12. Cotton, P. B. (1982) Duodenoscopic placement of biliary prostheses to relieve malignant obstructive jaundice. *Br. J. Surg.*, **69**, 501–3.
13. Safrany, L., Schott, B., Krause, S. *et al.* (1982) Endoskopische transpapilläre Gallengangsdrainage bei tumorbedingten Verschlussikterus. *Dtsch. Med. Wschr.*, **107**, 1867–71.
14. Huibregtse, K., Haverkamp, H. J., Hoogland, M. N. *et al.* (1981) A new instrument for cleaning and disinfection of fiberendoscopes. *Acta Endosc.*, **11**, 363–7.

Section D

RECENT ADVANCES IN INFLAMMATORY BOWEL DISEASE

21

Colonoscopy in the management of Crohn's disease

M. G. W. KETTLEWELL and P. H. HARPER

INTRODUCTION

Colonoscopy has been in general use for less than a decade and enthusiasts have been quick to experiment with the technique and to extend its useful role. However, as with any new techniques, colonoscopy has also been used indiscriminately out of curiosity, adding little to the management of some patients at the cost of some discomfort and a small risk of complications. Nonetheless recent experience has produced sufficient information to clarify the role of colonoscopy in Crohn's disease. It is therefore our intention to put colonoscopy in perspective in the management of patients with this disease. Over the last six years Crohn's disease has accounted for only 13% of all colonoscopies at Oxford despite a major interest in the disease.

DIAGNOSIS

There are numerous indications for colonoscopy in Crohn's disease and the main ones are summarized in Table 21.1. Endoscopy has replaced radiology and become the first line of investigation in the diagnosis of most oesophageal, gastric and duodenal diseases but at present it definitely plays a subordinate role in Crohn's disease of the small and large intestine. Good double contrast studies, with relaxation, remain the first choice for diagnosis and surveying the extent of the disease and the small bowel intubation examination, which gives far more definition and information, has superseded the standard small bowel follow through [1]. This increased diagnostic yield justifies the slightly more invasive technique. Colonoscopy is used only a third as often as radiological studies for

Table 21.1 Indications for colonoscopy in Crohn's disease

1) Diagnostic
2) Assessment of:
(a) Filling defects
(b) 'Strictures'
(c) Disease activity
3) Aid to surgery
4) Cancer surveillance
5) Research

Table 21.2 Colonoscopy for Crohn's disease in Oxford

Diagnostic	45.1%
(a) Definite +ve or −ve	31.7%
(b) Possible	13.4%
Disease assessment	54.9%
(a) Bowel in continuity	32.3%
(b) Split ileostomy	22.6%

Crohn's disease in Oxford, and of these endoscopies 45.5% have been diagnostic (Table 21.2). The main indication for diagnostic colonoscopy is in cases where good radiology has failed to provide a positive diagnosis and when the clinical index of suspicion of Crohn's disease is high, or if the radiological appearances are only suggestive of Crohn's. For example endoscopy is most valuable if the radiographs only show thickened folds (Fig. 21.1), or possible aphthous ulcers (Fig. 21.2). The former is a non-specific sign which occurs in early Crohn's disease while the latter may be an artefact due to uneven barium coating of the mucosa. Colonoscopy and biopsy is again valuable if the radiograph has identified a definite abnormality but the diagnosis is not clear.

A number of classical endoscopic appearances of Crohn's disease have been described (see below) but in spite of this a diagnosis is not always possible on macroscopic appearances alone, partly because these diagnostic features are not always present, and partly because there is considerable overlap with other inflammatory diseases. Ulcerative colitis in particular may be confused with Crohn's colitis since many of the endoscopic features are common to both diseases [2]. Similarly Crohn's ileitis may be mistaken for *Yersinia* infection or ileocaecal tuberculosis. Jejunal giardiasis may also mimic mild Crohn's disease. Although 45.1% of our colonoscopies were diagnostic, the macroscopic appearances allowed a confident diagnosis of Crohn's disease in only 70% of them. In the remaining 30% there were no diagnostic features even though the intestine was inflamed and abnormal. In these cases histological examination of biopsy specimens was required.

The great advantage of endoscopy is that numerous biopsies can be taken, but

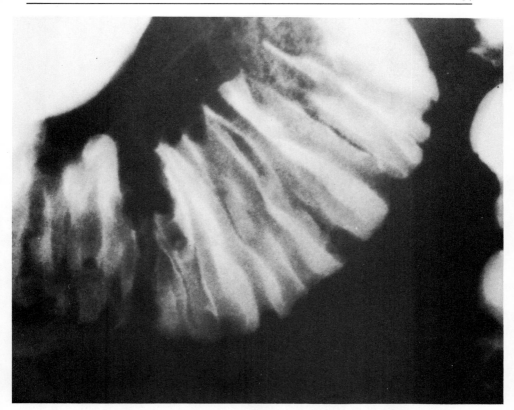

Fig. 21.1 A small bowel barium examination illustrating thickened valvulae coniventes, the earliest but non-specific radiological sign of Crohn's disease. (Reproduced with permission from the Editor of *Clinical Radiology*.)

these are small and predictably histologists often have difficulty distinguishing Crohn's from ulcerative colitis with confidence. In our experience Crohn's granulomas are uncommon in biopsy material which is also the experience of a number of others [2, 3, 4]. Some others however have found granulomas to be common [5]. The diagnostic yield may be increased by biopsing whole aphthous ulcers, taking deep bites of the edges of larger ulcers and also taking numerous biopsies not only of specific lesions but also serially throughout the bowel. As the diagnostic rate of malignancy in gastric ulcers increases with the number of biopsies so does the likelihood of diagnosing Crohn's disease. The patchy nature of the inflammation histologically and endoscopically is an important distinguishing feature from the uniformity of ulcerative colitis.

The discussion of whether radiology or colonoscopy is pre-eminent and which investigation provides the greater yield of useful information is essentially sterile. Both methods are valuable but they are complementary since the perspective of each is so totally different. The yield of each investigation is therefore additive.

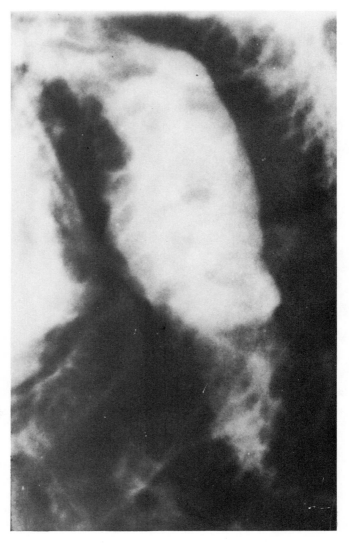

Fig. 21.2 A small bowel barium examination in a patient with ileal Crohn's disease illustrating aphthous ulceration. (Reproduced with permission from the Editor of *Clinical Radiology*.)

ASSESSMENT OF DISEASE

Filling defects

Cobblestoning and pseudopolyps, occasionally of giant proportions, are quite common in Crohn's colitis. Inflammatory polyps, asymmetrical scarring and distortion of the bowel wall are also hallmarks of Crohn's disease. All these features may show up as filling defects on radiographs in patients with known or suspected Crohn's disease. Since Crohn's as well as ulcerative colitis carries an increased risk of malignancy [6, 7] it is wise to examine any radiological lesion which could be neoplastic in order to obtain biopsies. Furthermore some pseudopolyps may be sufficiently large to cause intestinal obstruction [2, 8] and if they are not too broad based may be removed with the diathermy snare. Caution is needed if the surrounding mucosa is inflamed because the eschar will not heal well. In any event histological exclusion of malignancy allows a more conservative approach to patients who all too often require operations for other manifestations of their disease.

Carcinoma of the colon may also masquerade as Crohn's disease even in young people, particularly if the tumour is diffuse and infiltrating. Failure to recognize this possibility may lead to tragedy.

Filling defects in the small bowel are less likely to be neoplastic, nevertheless isolated and discrete lesions at either end of the small bowel should be inspected and biopsied endoscopically.

Strictures

There are two main reasons for endoscoping patients with strictures seen radiologically. Firstly to exclude the infiltrative, stenosing carcinoma of the colon. The incidence of carcinoma in long standing total ulcerative colitis is a little over 3% [7] and this increased risk is generally recognized. While the risk may be greater in ulcerative colitis than Crohn's disease there is increasing evidence that Crohn's patients are at greater risk of malignancy than the normal population [6], particularly in defunctioned small bowel [9]. The type of colonic cancer appears to be similar in both diseases. It is difficult to distinguish benign from malignant strictures on the macroscopic appearances, therefore it is necessary to take numerous biopsies of the stricture, particularly of both ends. While most strictures are benign [10] any which are unyielding, have a shelved edge, or are friable are likely to be malignant and should be treated as such [11].

The second reason for examining a stricture is to assess its lumen and therefore the degree of obstruction. Crohn's strictures are either inflammatory and symmetrical, or fibrotic and scarred when they are often asymmetrical. The soft inflammatory stricture may well resolve on treatment and since colicky abdominal pain and diarrhoea are common in Crohn's disease it is important to decide whether the symptoms are due to inflammation or obstruction. What appears narrow on a radiograph, particularly with conventional follow through examinations, may not be obstructing and may easily yield to the endoscope. Furthermore strictures which are sufficiently pliable to allow passage of the colonoscope are unlikely to need resection for fear of obstruction, particularly if they are in the ileum or right colon where the faeces is liquid. Small bowel strictures seldom need inspection if the intubation radiological examination has been used because the rapid infusion of barium into the small bowel distends it and demonstrates obstruction to the passage of barium.

It is possible to use, and worth considering the Eder–Puestow dilators to dilate short strictures of the sigmoid colon and upper rectum. The technique is safe if performed under radiological control and we have used this method to dilate three colonic strictures, one of which was due to Crohn's disease.

Assessment of disease extent and activity

Radiology undoubtedly provides the best overall estimate of the extent of disease throughout the whole intestine but endoscopy has shown repeatedly that obvious disease extends well beyond the radiological limits [12, 13]. Furthermore biopsy of endoscopically normal bowel shows that microscopic disease extends further still [14, 15]. Colonoscopy and ileoscopy are therefore useful in patients whose symptoms are not in proportion to the radiological estimate of disease. In cases which are iller than might be expected from radiographs, endoscopy and biopsy is likely to show that the disease is far more extensive.

Endoscopy also provides a clearer impression of disease activity than radiographs. Radiologically mild disease may in fact be severely inflamed. Conversely radiologically severe disease may be quiescent and the endoscopic features of inflammation absent despite marked distortion of the bowel.

Endoscopic assessment of disease extent and severity is particularly valuable after resection. Recurrent diarrhoea or pain after resection of the terminal ileum and caecum is a familiar problem. In these cases colonoscopy with ileal intubation will clarify whether the symptoms are due to recurrent Crohn's disease or failure of bile salt absorption.

CANCER AND DYSPLASIA

Colonoscopic surveillance of patients with long standing total ulcerative colitis is now well established because of the increased risk of cancer [13]. Crohn's disease also appears to have an increased risk of malignancy [6] and so a case can be advanced to endoscope the accessible intestine of patients with long standing Crohn's even if the precise risk is not known.

RESEARCH

The ability to take target biopsies repeatedly makes endoscopy an important research tool in the quest of a solution to Crohn's disease. Some of the ideas offered illustrate the wide range of possibilities in this fascinating condition. The patchy distribution, variability in inflammation, and asymmetry compared to ulcerative colitis raises many questions about the inflammatory process and its progression. Linear ulcers are nearly always on the mesenteric side of the bowel while aphthous ulcers are evenly spread around the circumference. Why this is so is far from clear but study of the immunopathology in endoscopic biopsies may provide some of the answers.

The operation of split ileostomy produces an immediate and dramatic clinical improvement in patients with severe Crohn's colitis [16]. Endoscopic and histological studies may clarify the role of faeces in the genesis or maintenance of Crohn's colitis.

Drug treatment often produces a marked clinical improvement in patients without producing a corresponding change in the endoscopic or microscopic appearances of the gut and this discrepancy requires further study.

TECHNIQUE

Crohn's disease lends itself to endoscopic imagination. Every portal of entry to the gastrointestinal tract is available for examination when the need arises. Conventional colonoscopy is probably most commonly used and the terminal 20–40 cm of ileum can also be examined in about 85% of patients. The Crohn's colon is often easier to examine than the normal because of scarring and shortening of the mesenteric side of the bowel. Otherwise the technique of intubation is no different from the normal. The proximal 20–50 cm of jejunum can readily be examined with the standard long colonoscope, appropriately cleaned, and introduced through the mouth. The remainder of the small bowel is extremely difficult to examine with any of the current endoscopes. However it can be examined during a laparotomy.

Colostomies, ileostomies and mucous fistulae also allow useful access to the intestine. While most colonoscopes can be inserted easily into a colostomy, ileostomies are often too narrow. The thinner paediatric gastoscopes however are excellent for examining 40–60 cm of small bowel. The same instruments are also most useful for colonoscoping small children with Crohn's.

Contraindications to endoscopy

While most patients with Crohn's disease can be endoscoped successfully and safely it is unwise to attempt endoscopy in any patient with fulminant colitis or gross colonic dilatation because of the risk of perforation. It is also unsafe to colonoscope anyone with severe abdominal pain or signs of peritonism for the same reason. Common sense dictates that colonoscopy is unnecessary and dangerous in any patient seriously ill with Crohn's disease.

Biopsy and histology

Because Crohn's disease is so patchy and asymmetrical both macroscopically and microscopically it is important to take numerous biopsies. The more biopsies there are the more likely the pathologist is to find the diagnostic granulomas [17]. The variation in the histology of biopsies from different parts of the gut is also diagnostic. The biopsies should be as generous as possible because most of the inflammation and granulomas are deep to the mucosa, and they should be of normal as well as inflamed mucosa. Aphthous ulcers in particular may yield granulomas.

Bowel preparation

Oral intubation of the jejunum requires no preparation other than a four-hour fast. The colon however needs meticulous preparation but many clinicians are afraid that vigorous preparation will exacerbate the colitis. Our experience is that progressively vigorous preparation for patients with both Crohn's disease and ulcerative colitis has not exacerbated the inflammation. Williams and Waye [13] have also shown that patients with inactive but extensive colitis will withstand vigorous preparation without ill effects.

Personal preference is wide but most people use some permutation of a liquid diet for 24–48 hours; a castor oil or magnesium purge, and one or two enemas or high colonic washouts. Alternatively an oral mannitol load (1 litre 10% mannitol) or whole gut saline irrigation has been advocated [18, 19]. Our preference is given in Table 21.3 and no concession is made for inactive colitis.

Patients with active colitis and diarrhoea do not need vigorous preparation and therefore it is unnecessary and unkind to use a strong purge. In these cases we use half the normal purgation and rely on the saline washouts to clear the faecal debris. It is worth remembering that phosphate enemas produce some mucosal oedema and erythema which may be mistaken for inflammatory bowel disease.

Complications

Complications are very rare in colonoscopy [20] and inflammatory bowel disease does not appear to increase the risks [21]. We have only had one complication in over 400 colonoscopies for inflammatory bowel disease of which 164 were for Crohn's disease. This patient with mild recurrent Crohn's disease was being investigated for recurrent blood loss and bled 1.5 l after colonoscopy and multiple biopsy.

Table 21.3 Bowel preparations for colonoscopy

Purge	Liquid diet	Enemas
Castor oil 45 ml	24 h	0.9% Saline 2 × 2 l
Picolax × 2	48 h	1 Phosphate

ENDOSCOPIC APPEARANCES OF CROHN'S DISEASE

The endoscopic appearances of Crohn's disease are fascinatingly varied both in distribution and extent. They also change with disease activity. The appearance of most diagnostic value is the variation in severity of disease throughout the bowel. Patches of severe, moderate, and mild disease are interspersed with each other as well as with normal mucosa to produce skip lesions. Within any field of view there may be active inflammation on one side of the bowel, usually the mesenteric side, with normal mucosa opposite. This endoscopic pleomorphism is the hallmark of Crohn's disease and is the most valuable diagnostic feature but occasionally the inflammation is uniform at least to the eye.

Active or inactive disease

The usual features of active inflammation are erythema, oedema with thickened mucosal folds, granularity, ulceration and friability with contact bleeding. The erythema and friability are less marked than ulcerative or ischaemic colitis but are nonetheless obvious. When the disease is inactive the appearances of the bowel depend to a large extent on the severity of the previous inflammation. For example the bowel may look quite normal after a mild attack but it is scarred and distorted after a severe attack. The normal mucosal folds are often lost and the mucosa looks atrophic. There may also be patches of granularity with loss of vascular pattern and if the scarring is severe then the intervening mucosa will be cobblestoned. Pseudopolyps persist in inactive disease but the surface epithelium does not show any of the characteristics of inflammation.

The endoscopic appearances of Crohn's disease of the colon and ileum are remarkably similar after making allowances for the structural differences in the two organs. The ileal mucosa is more velvety than the colonic mucosa and because it is thicker there is no submucosal vascular pattern. Ileal mucosal folds are more prominent than colonic haustra. The distribution of aphthous ulcers is however similar in both ileum and colon. The characteristic longitudinal ulcers are usually confined to the mesenteric border of the ileum as well as the colon (Fig. 21.3).

Strictures, as distinct from radiologically narrow areas in the small bowel are often short and abrupt with the cicatrix spreading round from the mesenteric side. In contrast colonic strictures are often longer and fusiform which implies confluent scarring. These distinctions are of course not absolute.

Active disease

Mild disease is characterized by oedema, thickening of the mucosal folds, some patchy granularity, red mucosal plaques [22] and aphthous ulcers (Table 21.4). The plaques and aphthous ulcers are evenly distributed round the circumference of the bowel but unevenly throughout its length. Some of these features, such as oedema, thickened folds, and even erythema are not specific for Crohn's disease and may be found in other conditions such as diverticulitis and giardiasis.

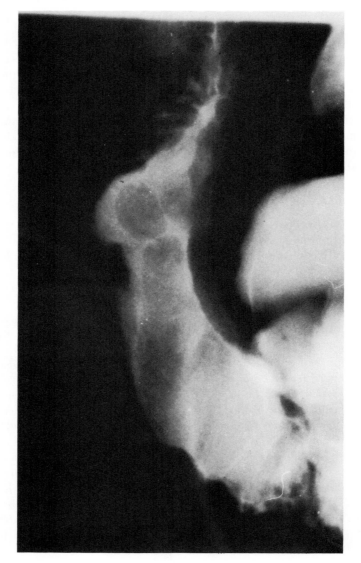

Fig. 21.3 A small bowel barium examination illustrating an extensive linear mesenteric ulcer of the ileum. The endoscopic appearances were of inactive disease. (Reproduced with permission from the Editor of *Clinical Radiology*.)

Erythema, linear mesenteric ulcers, serpiginous ulcers and cobblestones are features of moderately severe inflammation. Severe Crohn's disease however has confluent ulceration with marked mucosal friability and contact bleeding. There may also be mucosal bridging and pseudopolyp formation and they are also severely inflamed.

Table 21.4 Endoscopic features of Crohn's disease

	Active	Inactive
Mild	Oedema Thickened folds Red plaques Aphthous ulcers	Normal
Moderate	Erythema Linear ulcers Serpiginous ulcers Cobblestones	Patchy atrophy Distortion mild Cobblestones
Severe	Erythema Friability Confluent ulcers Bridging Pseudopolyps	Distortion gross Scarring Strictures Pseudopolyps

DIFFERENTIAL DIAGNOSIS

Ulcerative colitis is the major differential diagnosis. Aphthous ulcers and cobblestones are very seldom seen in ulcerative colitis and are therefore important points of distinction but many of the other features are common to both diseases [2]. The geographic pattern and pleomorphism are usually sufficient to distinguish the two. Ulcerative colitis is much more uniform and the inflammation tends to increase towards the rectum although topical steroids may produce some rectal sparing. Similarly, few histological features other than granulomas are unique to either disease [2] and so variability of the inflammation favours Crohn's disease. Diverticulitis and Crohn's colitis may coexist in the sigmoid colon but the endoscopic features of diverticulitis alone are thickened folds, oedema, narrowing of the lumen, erythema and mucosal petaechae but no ulceration.

Tuberculous ileocolitis is very difficult to distinguish from Crohn's endoscopically and histology is often unhelpful because acid-fast bacilli and caseation are seldom seen on biopsies [23, 24]. Tuberculosis should therefore be considered in any patient from countries where the disease is endemic.

Jejunal giardiasis produces oedema and erythema like Crohn's but the organisms are readily seen on biopsies.

Yersinia infections cause a uniform small haemorrhagic ulceration in the colon [25] and granularity and erythema in the terminal ileum.

Acute ischaemic colitis has a cyanotic mucosa which is more or less friable and haemorrhagic. The histological features are usually obvious [26]. Bowel preparation rarely produces a colitis. This has occurred three times in our experience when hypertonic saline was used accidently for the washouts. The appearances were mistaken for Crohn's disease initially because the colitis was patchy with small haemorrhagic ulcers which were ischaemic histologically.

Irradiation enteritis usually appears as an atrophic but friable mucosa often with strictures. There may also be ulceration but biopsies confirm the radiation endarteritis and ischaemia.

Patients with the Irritable Colon Syndrome are often colonoscoped and the mucosa is always normal but the colon is often crenated and puckered. It may also be extremely active and irritable inspite of sedation.

CONCLUSION

Colonoscopy with intubation of the terminal ileum or examination of the proximal jejunum with a colonoscope are relatively easy and trouble-free investigations which provide valuable information in a quarter to a third of patients with Crohn's disease. The technique has validated the radiological signs of mild Crohn's disease and it is particularly useful for assessing the extent and activity of the disease.

REFERENCES

1. Nolan, D. J. (1981) Barium examination of the small intestine: progress report. *Gut*, **22**, 682–94.
2. Waye, J. D. (1980) Endoscopy in inflammatory bowel disease. *Clin. Gastroenterol.*, **9**, 279–96.
3. McGovern, V. J. and Goulston, S. J. M. (1968) Crohn's disease of the colon. *Gut*, **9**, 164–76.
4. Geboes, K., Desmet, V. J., De Wolf-Peeters, C. and Vantrappen, G. (1978) The value of endoscopic biopsies in the diagnosis of Crohn's disease. *Am. J. Proctol.*, **29**, 21–8.
5. Lux, G., Fruhmorgen, P., Phillip, J. and Zeus, J. (1978) Diagnosis of inflammatory diseases of the colon. *Endoscopy*, **10**, 279–84.
6. Gyde, S. N., Prior, P., Macartney, J. C. *et al.* (1980) Malignancy in Crohn's disease. *Gut*, **21**, 1024–9.
7. Whelan, G. (1980) Cancer risk in ulcerative colitis: why are results in the literature so varied? *Clin. Gastroenterol.*, **9**, 469–76.
8. Di Febo, G., Gizzi, G. and Cappello, I. P. (1981) Unusual case of colonic sub-obstruction by giant pseudopolyposis in Crohn's colitis. *Endoscopy*, **13**, 90–2.
9. Greenstein, A. J., Sacher, D., Pucillo, A. *et al.* (1978) Cancer in Crohn's disease after diversionary surgery. *Am. J. Surg.*, **135**, 86–90.
10. Hunt, R. H., Teague, R. H., Swarbrick, E. T. and Williams, C. B. (1975) Colonoscopy in the management of colonic strictures. *Br. Med. J.*, **2**, 360–1.
11. Cook, M. G. and Goligher, J. C. (1975) Carcinoma and epithelial dysplasia complicating ulcerative colitis. *Gastroenterology*, **68**, 1127–36.
12. Geboes, K. and Vantrappen, G. (1975) The value of colonoscopy in the diagnosis of Crohn's disease. *Gastrointest. Endosc.*, **22**, 18–23.
13. Williams, C. B. and Waye, J. D. (1978) Colonoscopy in inflammatory bowel disease. *Clin. Gastroenterol.*, **7**, 701–17.

14. Hogan, W. J., Hensley, G. T. and Geenan, J. E. (1980) Endoscopic evaluation of inflammatory bowel disease. *Med. Clin. N. Am.*, **64**. 1083–102.
15. Mitros, F. A. (1980) The biopsy in evaluating patients with inflammatory bowel disease. *Med. Clin. N. Am.*, **64**, 1037–57.
16. Harper, P. H., Truelove, S. C., Lee, E. C. G., Kettlewell, M. G. W. and Jewell, D. P. (1982) Split ileostomy and ileocolostomy for Crohn's disease of the colon and ulcerative colitis: a 20 year survey. *Gut*, **24**, 106–13.
17. Chambers, T. J. and Morson, B. C. (1980) Large bowel biopsy in the diagnosis of inflammatory bowel disease, *Invest. Cell Pathol.*, **2**, 159–73.
18. Hewitt, J., Reeve, J. and Rigby, J. (1973) Whole-gut irrigation in preparation for large-bowel surgery. *Lancet*, **ii**, 337–40.
19. Donovan, I. A., Arabi, Y., Keighley, M. R. B. and Alexander-Williams, J. (1980) Modification of the physiological disturbances produced by whole gut irrigation by preliminary mannitol administration. *Br. J. Surg.*, **67**, 138–9.
20. Overholt, B. F. (1975) Colonoscopy: a review. *Gastroenterology*, **68**, 1308–20.
21. Smith, L. E. (1976) Complications of colonoscopy and polypectomy. *Dis. Colon Rectum*, **19**, 407–12.
22. Watier, A., Devroede, G., Perey, B. *et al.* (1981) Small erythematous plaques: an endoscopic sign of Crohn's disease. *Gut*, **21**, 835–9.
23. Watanabe, H., Hiwatashi, N. and Goto, Y. (1979) Biopsy under direct vision for the diagnosis of Crohn's disease. *Tohuku J. Exp. Med.*, **129**, 1–8.
24. Bretholtz, A., Stasser, H. and Knoblauch, M. (1978) Endoscopic diagnosis of ileocaecal tuberculosis. *Gastrointest. Endosc.*, **26**, 250–1.
25. Vantrappen, G., Agg, H. O., Ponette, E., Geboes, K. and Bertrand, P. (1977) Yersinia enteritis and enterocolitis: gastroenterological aspects. *Gastroenterology*, **72**, 220–7.
26. Whitehead, R. (1979) *Mucosal Biopsy of the Gastrointestinal Tract*, (2nd edn), W. B. Saunders Co., Philadelphia, pp. 152–96.

22

Colonoscopy and the indications for surgery in ulcerative colitis

JEROME D. WAYE and SANFORD BRAUNFELD

Ulcerative colitis is an inflammatory disease of unknown aetiology which affects the large intestine. Surgical extirpation of the colon provides the patient with a permanent cure of this disease [1]. In spite of the ability to eradicate ulcerative colitis completely by surgical means, only 15–20% [2] of patients with ulcerative colitis have surgical intervention. A major reason for the low surgery rate is undoubtedly that the end result is usually a permanent ileostomy following total colectomy. Due to abhorrence of an ileostomy, physicians and patients together brave serious complications and even death to preserve normal defaecatory function. Dealing with an acutely ill patient requires careful clinical observation, with ongoing assessment frequently necessitating hour-to-hour re-evaluation and continuous monitoring by members of the medical/surgical team; colonoscopy does not have a role in the overall evaluation and eventual therapy of such patients, nor does endoscopy contribute to the decision for surgery in the patient whose disease progresses inexorably, despite the judicious use of drugs, such as corticosteroids, and parenteral nutrition. In the majority of patients, the decision for surgery is based on the sudden onset of clinical factors which arise as complications of the disease, such as uncontrolled haemorrhage, free or confined perforation of the bowel, and toxic megacolon. In the non-emergency patient, the decision for surgery is a clinical judgment based on a complex integration of several weighted parameters, most of which are poorly measured but include response to therapy and the rate of progress of the total disease process. Other complications of ulcerative colitis, such as growth retardation and the extraintestinal manifestations, including ocular involvement, arthritis, pyoderma gangrenosum and hepatic abnormalities, must be handled from a multidisciplinary approach, none of which involves colonoscopy. Of the total number of ulcerative colitis patients requiring surgery, in only a few does colonoscopy offer definitive assistance in reaching a surgical decision.

During the 15 years since colonoscopy was first introduced, a well-accepted set of general indications has developed. Within the area of inflammatory bowel disease, a specific subset of usage can be identified (Table 22.1). Most patients with inflammatory bowel disease will live through the entire span of their illness without ever requiring colonoscopic evaluation. In patients with ulcerative colitis, the greatest benefit of colonoscopy occurs when specific goals can be identified that may be achieved with endoscopy; this would prevent subjecting patients with inflammatory bowel disease to procedures which may be unnecessary.

Colonoscopy may directly influence the decision for surgery during the course of ulcerative colitis in the following manner:

(a) Confirmation of diagnosis (ulcerative colitis *vs.* Crohn's disease)
(b) Evaluation of a filling defect on barium enema radiological examination
(c) Evaluation of a colonic stricture
(d) Discovery of premalignant changes in the colon
(e) Postoperative evaluation of a rectal segment following total colectomy

The determination of the extent of disease is rarely considered a factor in the ultimate decision for surgery, unless the distal large bowel is the only area affected. In this circumstance, estimation of the length of involved bowel can usually be ascertained by sigmoidoscopy and barium enema radiological examination, with realization that the group of patients in whom the barium enema may fail to delineate the full extent of mucosal involvement have relatively mild proximal disease [3], and are rarely considered as surgical problems.

The correct diagnosis of the type of colitis may not be achieved in spite of the completion of a battery of tests, examinations and even sigmoidoscopically obtained biopsy material. The surgical approach to the patient with ulcerative colitis may be quite different than for the patient with Crohn's disease, and special efforts must be directed toward establishing the correct diagnosis when surgery is being contemplated. Although modern radiological techniques with double contrast can often demonstrate the small aphthous ulcers in Crohn's disease, these may not be seen on every examination, and direct endoscopic visualization of the colonic mucosa may be required to make the differential diagnosis.

Whenever colonoscopy is indicated during the course of ulcerative colitis, complete intubation of the entire large bowel is desirable. If, however, the

Table 22.1 Indications for colonoscopy in ulcerative colitis

Differential diagnosis
Identification of radiographic abnormalities
 Mass lesions
 Stricture
Examination of stomas
Examination of retained rectal segment
Determination of extent of disease
Screening for premalignant and malignant features

predetermined goal of colonoscopy can be achieved by a partial examination, it may be wise to discontinue the procedure rather than risk a perforation in a markedly inflamed bowel during vigorous, but misguided, attempts to perform a total colonoscopy. When the indication for an examination is determination of cancer or precancer, a total endoscopy is desired, whereas a complete colonic inspection may not be necessary for the evaluation of a stricture or other radiographic abnormality. When an attempt is made to establish the proper differential diagnosis by colonoscopy, the examination may be terminated at any point when the endoscopist has been able to reach a definite conclusion. In a personal series of consecutive examinations in 289 patients with inflammatory bowel disease, endoscopy to the caecum was performed in 94% of patients with ulcerative colitis and in 74% of patients with Crohn's disease. The higher degree of endoscopy in patients with ulcerative colitis reflects the need for total colon evaluation in searching for malignancy in these patients. Inspection of the entire colon is both desirable and feasible in the majority of these patients; a recent article from Sweden [4] reported a 92% rate of complete colonoscopy. When total colonoscopy is not accomplished in these patients, the reason is either a stricture or poor preparation of the colon, whereas in the patient with Crohn's disease cessation of the examination is most frequently due to severity of the inflammatory process, with large, deep ulcerations.

Visual criteria may be more useful in rendering the correct differential diagnosis than a review of biopsy material, since a specific conclusion is rarely possible on the basis of the small specimens obtained. The incidence of granulomas found during colonoscopic tissue sampling is low and varies from observer to observer. Although granulomas are the pathognomonic histopathological feature in patients with granulomatous colitis, their absence on biopsy does not increase the probability of ulcerative colitis as a true diagnosis, since only 3% of patients at the Mount Sinai Hospital with the clinical diagnosis of Crohn's disease have this finding on tissue biopsy samples gathered colonoscopically. The literature on granuloma incidence presents a wide range of variability [5, 6, 7], probably related to the type of patients seen, since aphthous ulcers seen in the course of Crohn's disease provide the highest yield of granulomas on biopsy. Patients endoscoped early in the course of inflammatory bowel disease at the time that these small ulcers are present will provide the highest yield of granulomas on biopsy examination. Once the ulcer enlarges beyond 2–5 cm in diameter, the probability of finding a granuloma diminishes. Other histopathological features are less specific, such as crypt abscesses, although considered a hallmark of ulcerative colitis, may be present in both ulcerative and granulomatous colitis but are less frequent in patients with Crohn's disease (Table 22.2). Upon reviewing pathology specimens on colonoscopically obtained biopsies from patients with inflammatory bowel disease, it is evident that the most common pathological finding is that of non-specific inflammatory infiltration with reports of 'acute and/or chronic inflammation' on several biopsy specimens. The astute pathologist may make the suggestion that the collective multiple biopsies are 'compatible with granulomatous colitis', or 'compatible

Table 22.2 Pathology reports on colonoscopic biopsies (in percent)

	Granulomatous colitis (88 patients)	Ulcerative colitis (146 patients)
Crypt abscess	13	25
Acute and/or chronic inflammation	92	90
Chronic inflammation with lymphoid follicle	5	5
Inflammation involves submucosa	7	4
Granulation tissue	11	6
Compatible with granulomatous colitis	10	—
Compatible with ulcerative colitis	1	15

with ulcerative colitis' by identifying the pattern of 'skip areas' or 'patchy inflammation' in granulomatous colitis as opposed to the distally increasing inflammation in ulcerative colitis. In contradistinctions to the unerring accuracy of the pathologist's diagnosis when provided with several grams of tissue or many centimetres of gut, the interpretation of these small superficial biopsy fragments is frequently aided by knowledge of the patient's clinical presentation. It is in the interpretation of endoscopic biopsy specimens that close cooperation must develop between the clinician and the pathologist.

Several gross pathological features are present in each type of inflammatory bowel disease that permit the trained endoscopist to differentiate accurately between ulcerative and granulomatous colitis [8]. Important factors are:

(a) *Pattern of involvement.* In ulcerative colitis, the rectum is usually involved, whereas it may or may not be affected in granulomatous disease. Patchy areas of involvement with erythema and ulcerations are common in patients with Crohn's disease, but the involvement with ulcerative colitis is usually contiguous and symmetrical from the rectum proximal to the point of cessation of disease. Granulomatous colitis frequently involves only the right colon, so that inflammation, ulcerations and mucosal irregularities seen in the proximal colon are strong evidence in favour of granulomatous colitis.

(b) *Mucosal involvement.* Early in the course of ulcerative colitis, the normal vascular pattern may be obscured by the diffuse erythema accompanying the inflammatory mucosal involvement. Surface trauma occurs easily from the passage of stool or from instrumentation, with punctate bleeding. Friability may be associated with another frequently described characteristic in ulcerative colitis termed granularity, caused by pinpoint ulcerations with surrounding mucosal oedema. The microulcerations and oedema produce an endoscopic appearance similar to that of wet sandpaper (granularity). Friability and diffuse erythema may also be present in Crohn's disease but usually occur late in the course of granulomatous colitis as opposed to their early appearance in ulcerative colitis. The mucosa in Crohn's disease usually has normal-appearing vascular patterns and is not involved diffusely. Because of the submucosal involvement in granulomatous colitis, broad, asymmetric nodulations may occur and produce the typical 'cobblestoning' characteristic of Crohn's disease but never present in ulcerative colitis.

(c) *Ulcerations in ulcerative colitis.* The ulcerations in ulcerative colitis always occur in areas of diffusely abnormal mucosa. If ulcerations are seen in segments of colon that appear otherwise normal, with an intact vascular pattern surrounding an ulceration, the diagnosis is definitely *not* ulcerative colitis. Small aphthous ulcerations are characteristic of Crohn's disease and are the earliest mucosal abnormality. As the disease progresses, the ulcers in granulomatous colitis become larger and longitudinally linear.

(d) *Similarities in inflammatory bowel disease.* Pseudopolyps may occur in both diseases and, at the Mount Sinai Hospital, are seen endoscopically in 30% of patients with Crohn's disease and 47% of patients with ulcerative colitis. The interhaustral septa are thickened and blunted in areas of involvement in both types of inflammatory bowel disease. It should be emphasized that, in the majority of patients with inflammatory bowel disease, the correct diagnosis is clear from the time of initial patient evaluation through information gathered from a thorough medical history, the proctosigmoidoscopic examination, and the barium enema. Colonoscopy is of limited usefulness in the differential diagnosis but adds yet another parameter to the total assessment of the patient.

The barium enema radiograph is properly considered to be the standard for evaluation of the entire colon in patients with ulcerative colitis. The radiological examination, in conjunction with regular clinical evaluation and periodic sigmoidiscopy, will provide an answer to almost all the diagnostic and therapeutic questions that occur during the patient's course of colitis. A few patients will require the addition of colonoscopy to the standard diagnostic procedures when a specific problem arises. One of the situations in which colonoscopy may be useful is in the investigation of a radiographically undiagnosed filling defect. Most filling defects in the well-prepared patient with ulcerative colitis are caused by pseudopolyps. These small polyps are readily identified on the roentgenographic examination and are rarely confused with more significant mass lesions, such as carcinoma of the colon. Although pseudopolyps are usually small (less than 7 mm in diameter) [9] and multiple, some may be not only solitary, but grow to several centimetres in diameter [10]. These large pseudopolyps, or a collection of small pseudopolyps, may obstruct or act as a nidus for intussusception of the colon. Biopsies from any portion of a pseudopolyp will establish its correct identity, since the histological characteristics reflect the pathogenesis of these polyps. Some pseudopolyps are composed of granulation tissue and may be associated with surface bleeding [11]. Other pseudopolyps may occur as a result of the abnormal growth of epithelial islands left intact by the ravaging ulcerative process around them; as the ulcerations heal, the regenerative epithelial islands may grow disproportionately to the growth rate of surrounding, re-epithelialized mucosa, resulting in the appearance of polypoid tags of mucosal tissue projecting into the colonic lumen. Pseudopolyps are usually sessile, smooth and glistening, with the widest portion at the base, and characteristically are taller than the base is wide (finger-shaped). This is in contradistinction to sessile adenomas in the non-colitic colon, which usually have a base broader in diameter than the height of the polyp. Pseudopolyps may be myriad and widely distributed throughout the colon and usually can be identified by visual inspection alone. Pseudopolyps do not have any malignant potential and, once identified as such, may safely be ignored. Those that cause bleeding may be resected endoscopically, but surgical resection is usually required for the collections of pseudopolyps responsible for intussusception. Biopsy of pseudopolyps is usually unnecessary [3], unless they are large (over 1 cm in diameter), have an irregular surface configuration, are friable or appear different in coloration from other pseudopolyps. These same features may also be associated with adenomas or carcinoma of the colon, and biopsy may be the only method of differentiation.

Adenomatous polyps can be present in the colitic bowel but rarely are identified as such with the colonoscope. The typical pedunculated, reddened adenoma so commonly encountered in the non-colitic colon is an infrequent occurrence in ulcerative colitis, with most adenomas having the appearance of pseudopolyps, and only biopsy may establish the correct diagnosis [12]. Adenomas may be removed endoscopically, although healing of any polypectomy site may be delayed when endoscopic resection is performed in an area of active inflammation.

Since adenomas have a premalignant potential, it is desirable to attempt their removal endoscopically, since colotomy and polypectomy is not a procedure well tolerated by the colitic colon. If abnormal cellular architecture is present in colonoscopic biopsy specimens, and the polyp is not amenable to colonoscopic removal, surgery must be contemplated when these adenomas are over 1.0 cm in diameter.

Colonic strictures are another indication for colonoscopy in the operative evaluation of patients with ulcerative colitis. A clinical axiom holds that a stricture in a patient with ulcerative colitis is carcinoma until proven otherwise. Colonoscopy is a tool with which all strictures identified radiographically should be evaluated to determine the proper indication for surgery. In spite of the clinical axiom, most strictures in the colitic bowel are benign, but, until proper evaluation is accomplished, the risk of missing a malignancy exists. Hunt et al. [13] demonstrated via colonoscopy that only 12.5% of strictures in patients with ulcerative colitis are associated with malignancy in their series of 24 patients. Grandqvist et al. [4] reported that no cancer was found on a similar evaluation of 14 patients. The benign narrowed segments may be due to cicatricial fibrosis or to the muscular spasm associated with a localized segment of inflammation. The proper evaluation of strictures requires direct visual inspection along with biopsies and brush cytology from within the strictured area. Most strictures can be intubated with the standard-sized colonoscope and will often become dilated by air insufflated for the endoscopic examination. It is frequent that a narrowed segment on barium enema radiological examination cannot be identified with the colonoscope due to a combination of air inflation and the inability to appreciate minor changes in luminal circumference due to the 'fisheye' wide-angle optics of modern endoscopes. An inflammatory stricture is concentric, can usually be intubated with the colonoscope, and is identified by the significant degree of inflammation both surrounding and within it. A fibrotic stricture, on the other hand, is usually quite narrow, has a web-like configuration, and may occur in a bowel segment with no evidence of adjacent inflammation.

Adequate characterization of a stricture requires more than visual inspection of the entire segment, including both ends and the inner aspect of the narrowed area. When a stricture cannot be intubated, a paediatric instrument may be used to advantage [14], especially if the segment is in the left colon. Even when the stricture can be intubated, it may be possible to miss a carcinoma within it [15] when the tumour tends to spread submucosally and have only a minor surface component. It is, therefore, important to obtain biopsy and brush cytology from both edges of a strictured segment, as well as from the middle of the narrowed segment. Strictures which are too narrow to be intubated with the standard or paediatric endoscope should be referred for surgery, since adequate colonoscopic inspection is not possible. Endoscopic features which may signal the presence of malignancy within a stricture are: rigidity of the edge, an eccentric lumen, or abrupt shelf-like margins. Caution must be exercised in the inspection of a stricture lest perforation occur, since the wall in inflammatory bowel disease is less resilient to stretch than that of the normal colon. The endoscopist must be prepared to terminate the examination when a stricture resists gentle attempts at intubation. There is no role for the use of the colonoscopic tip as a dilating probe in colonic strictures occurring in ulcerative colitis.

The tendency for patients with ulcerative colitis to develop colon carcinoma at a much greater rate than occurs in the general population is a concern that requires prompt and thorough investigation of radiographic abnormalities in this group of patients. Carcinoma of the large bowel has a different pathogenesis in the patient with ulcerative colitis than in the non-colitic colon. There is considerable evidence that the adenoma–carcinoma sequence is the usual pathway for development of carcinoma of the 'normal' colon [16]. This concept of carcinoma development involves a focus of uncontrolled cellular growth on the periphery of the mucosal surface of an adenoma; as the cells proliferate without regulation, invasion into the stroma of the adenoma occurs, and over a length of time a typical bulky carcinoma develops. In the colitic colon, however, the diffuse inflammatory process which involves the mucosal surface appears to provoke the subsequent development of the abnormal cellular growth patterns, irrespective of the degree of colitic activity. Thus, the involved length of colon is at risk for the development of carcinoma, which may begin in quiescent segments of the colon containing areas of apparently healed mucosa, with malignancy arising from a previously non-polypoid, flat portion of the colon wall. Morson's studies [17] of carcinogenesis in the colitic colon have greatly enhanced both the understanding of and the approach to malignancy in ulcerative colitis. The earliest histological abnormality in the sequence of carcinoma development in the colitic colon is epithelial dysplasia, reflecting the abnormal cellular development [18]. Since the entire colon is at risk in the patient with universal, long-standing ulcerative colitis (over eight years' duration), the presence of dysplasia in one area is a marker of a tendency for that particular colon to harbour abnormal cellular development. Riddell and Morson [19] have emphasized the patchy nature of dysplasia and the need to take multiple biopsies throughout the colon to prevent missing dysplastic areas. Recent articles [20, 21] have refuted the previous view [22] that proximal dysplasia may occur as an isolated finding in one-third of patients with ulcerative colitis and dysplasia. If it is true that all patients with dysplasia in the proximal colon also have dysplasia on rectal biopsy [20, 21], there is no role for colonoscopy in the search for dysplasia. However, Riddell [23] has demonstrated that patches of dysplasia are relatively small and rarely exceed 5 cm in diameter, with 1–2 cm being the usual area of dysplastic involvement. Therefore, multiple biopsies must be obtained so that dysplastic changes are not missed. These are currently being taken via colonoscopy at 10–15 cm distances, which though not the most optimal for discovery of dysplastic changes, must be accepted as adequate because of the limitations imposed on obtaining more specimens both by the patient's tolerance of the procedure, and by the patience of the endoscopist.

Dysplasia is usually multifocal and its discovery in one segment is frequently associated with similar dysplastic changes in another, perhaps remote area of the colon at risk; its presence on biopsy should be a warning to the clinician that other segments in that large bowel are capable of developing or harbouring invasive carcinoma, the next step in the dysplasia sequence.

Many studies in the literature have confirmed Morson's [17] original findings on the importance of dysplasia in patients with universal, long-standing ulcerative colitis. Dysplasia can be a useful marker for the identification of colitis patients at ultra-high risk for the development of carcinoma. Following colonic resection for carcinoma of the colon, it has been shown by the clinical pathologist that 80% [21, 24] to 88% [22] of patients have dysplasia in other segments of the colitic colon. In spite of the high correlation of dysplasia found in ulcerative colitis patients who have a known cancer, in a review of the literature concerning dysplasia [25], this finding was reported in only 5.7% of rectal biopsies in patients with ulcerative colitis, and one-third of these patients had carcinoma of the colon. Dysplasia on rectal biopsy, therefore, results in a high yield (33%) of associated cancer. Although many of the previous reports were based on data obtained from resected colon specimens, several authors alluded to the potential usefulness of colonoscopy in the follow-up of the colitic patient. In order to assess the role of colonoscopy in patients with long-standing ulcerative colitis, a prospective study was initiated for gathering information on the colonoscopic follow-up of patients with long-standing universal ulcerative colitis. Up until July, 1980, 169 patients had colonoscopic examinations during the course of their ulcerative colitis disease. Two hundred and nineteen colonoscopies were performed in this group of patients, with 1149 biopsies obtained during the course of colonoscopy. Prior to the beginning of the study, it was apparent that many patients were being evaluated by colonoscopy for specific *diagnostic* problems that had developed during the course of their ulcerative colitis, such as: stricture, a mass lesion on radiology, change in the nature of symptoms, etc. Another group of patients could be identified in whom there were no specific complaints and in whom no reason for the endoscopic examination was present, except for surveillance of the colon for evidence of precancer. This group of patients could be readily separated out and are called the *surveillance* group [26]. In this study, 115 patients were evaluated for diagnostic purposes, and 54 patients were seen for endoscopic surveillance (Table 22.3). The number of biopsies per colon for surveillance purposes has gradually increased from 3.6% in 1975 to 8.0% in 1979. Since 1978, eight or more biopsies have been obtained in every patient undergoing surveillance colonoscopy. In any investigation involving ulcerative colitis and dysplasia, it is of paramount importance to separate clearly patients into the two major categories of diagnostic and surveillance groups. Results of all studies should be clearly identified as to whether the patients belong to one category or the other. If results are not separated, the true importance of surveillance studies involving dysplasia cannot be evaluated; patients whose biopsies are obtained during the investigation of a radiographically identified mass or stricture may be expected to have an incidence of dysplasia greater than the patients whose examinations were performed strictly for surveillance purposes.

In the diagnostic group of 115 patients (Table 22.4), 10 patients were found to have dysplasia. In this group, nine had no cancer on follow-up (two were operated upon). One patient with dysplasia had a carcinoma found at surgery (within a stricture). Six patients had a biopsy diagnosis of carcinoma but had no dysplasia on colonoscopic biopsies throughout the remainder of their colon. In this

Table 22.3 Colonoscopy in ulcerative colitis

	Total	Diagnostic	Surveillance
Patients	169	115	54
Colonoscopies	219	135	84
Biopsies	1149		

Table 22.4 Diagnostic group (115 patients), patients with dysplasia and/or cancer in ulcerative colitis

Dysplasia	Cancer
9	0
1	1
0	6

diagnostic group, seven patients, therefore, had carcinoma, and in only one was dysplasia reported on colonoscopic biopsy.

In the surveillance group, an additional nine patients have been studied since 1980 (Table 22.5). A total of 63 patients were entered in this group; five had the biopsy finding of dysplasia. Of these, four patients have been followed for up to three years and have not been found to have carcinoma. One patient with dysplasia was found during that same examination to have another biopsy from a flat mucosal segment which was reported as cancer. One other patient had the biopsy diagnosis of carcinoma, but no evidence of dysplasia in the other colonoscopic biopsies was present throughout the colon. Both patients in whom carcinoma was found in this surveillance group did not have any mass lesions which directed the biopsy to a specific area; both were discovered on routine multiple biopsy examinations. In this series, therefore, five out of 63 patients in the surveillance group had dysplasia (8%). One of five patients who had dysplasia on colonoscopic biopsy also had a simultaneous biopsy report of a focus of carcinoma. A total of two carcinomas (one of which had associated dysplasia) were found on colonoscopic biopsy in this surveillance, an incidence of 3% of patients having carcinoma discovered on routine colonoscopic biopsy.

The number of patients in this series is small but does indicate that multiple random biopsies may be as worthwhile in the discovery of carcinoma of the colon as is the finding of dysplasia, with one patient in the surveillance group found to have carcinoma with and another without associated dysplasia. None of the patients in whom dysplasia alone was found on colonoscopic biopsy have developed cancer, but the follow-up period is limited. There are a few reports that deal with surveillance colonoscopy and dysplasia, either directly or permit some comparative data to be gleaned from them. Fuson et al. [27] from the Cleveland Clinic have developed similar categories of surveillance colonoscopy and diagnostic colonoscopy in reporting their patients being followed for ulcerative colitis. They feel, as do we, that this is an important distinction. In Table 22.6 are listed the data contained in the seven studies (including the currently reported series) of colonoscopy and surveillance evaluation of patients with chronic universal ulcerative colitis [4, 21, 27–30]. The group from Leeds [28] followed 43 patients in their surveillance group, of whom nine had dysplasia. In their series, two patients found to have dysplasia were subsequently discovered to have carcinoma in the colon. Only two of the nine patients with dysplasia had this finding in the rectum.

Table 22.5 Surveillance group (63 patients), patients with dysplasia and/or cancer in ulcerative colitis

	Dysplasia	Cancer
	4	0
	1	1
	0	1

Table 22.6 Prospective colonoscopic surveillance in ulcerative colitis (479 patients)

	No. patients	No. patients with dysplasia	% Dysplasia	No. patients with dysplasia leading to cancer discovery	Dysplasia and cancer simultaneously	Cancer without dysplasia
Blackstone et al. [30]	66	6	9	1	0	0
Dickinson et al. [28]	43	9	20	2	0	0
Fuson et al. [27]	49	8	16	1	0	3
Grandqvist et al. [4]	150	12	8	1	0	0
Lennard-Jones et al. [29]	72 (CF)*	7	—	2	0	0
Nugent et al. [21]	36	8	22	2	0	0
Waye and Braunfeld	63	5	8	0	1	1

* Patients examined in the 'colonoscopy era'.

The total number of patients in the surveillance group followed by Lennard-Jones *et al.* [29] cannot be ascertained, since diagnostic and surveillance endoscopies were listed together. However, from a graphic presentation in their article, it is evident that seven patients in the surveillance category had dysplasia on colonoscopy, and, of these, two were found to have carcinoma at subsequent operation. Nugent *et al.* [21] reported on 36 patients undergoing colonoscopic surveillance, eight of whom had dysplasia. Of these, two had carcinoma at operation. Fuson *et al.* [27] followed 49 patients of whom eight had dysplasia. One of the patients with dysplasia was found at operation to have carcinoma, and in two additional patients carcinoma was reported to be present on biopsy specimens taken during the course of surveillance colonoscopy. One other patient had the biopsy diagnosis of a tubulovillous adenoma which, at surgery, was found to contain carcinoma. Therefore, four patients in the Cleveland Clinic group [27] were found to have carcinoma, only one of which was discovered because of the biopsy finding of dysplasia on colonoscopy. Blackstone *et al.* [30] performed surveillance examinations in 66 patients. Six patients in this group had dysplasia on colonoscopic biopsies directed at a specific lesion or mass in the colon. Of these six, one patient was found to have carcinoma at surgery. The total number of patients having dysplasia in their surveillance group is not possible to calculate, since they also report that, in their total group, only one of 27 patients who had dysplasia on biopsies of flat colonic mucosa was found to have a subsequent carcinoma. The proportion of these 27 patients with dysplasia who were in the surveillance group versus the diagnostic group was not listed. Blackstone *et al.* [30] found a high incidence of dysplasia and associated cancer in patients being investigated because of the radiographic identification of a mass or lesion. However, these were clearly not patients in the surveillance group. In the current series (Table 22.4) presented herein, the diagnostic group had a high yield of biopsy-proven carcinoma rather than dysplasia associated with a nearby malignancy. Our data are in agreement with the Blackstone study, in that the incidence of carcinoma is quite low when dysplasia was found in flat segments of the mucosa (one out of 27 patients), and relatively low when dysplasia was found on the surface of a mass or lesion in the surveillance group of patients (one out of six patients).

In addition to the 63 patients in our personal series, there have been 416 patients reported in the literature with chronic ulcerative colitis for over eight years' duration who could be included in a surveillance group (Table 22.6). A total of 479 patients have had surveillance colonoscopy, in 55 of whom dysplasia was found. The incidence of reported dysplasia in the surveillance group ranges from 8–22%, with a mean of 11%, suggesting that 1/10 patients in the high-risk group will, on colonoscopic biopsy, be found to have dysplasia. Fourteen patients in this surveillance group had cancer (an incidence of cancer/total patients of $14/479 = 3.0\%$), with nine carcinomas discovered as a result of investigation because of the previous diagnosis of dysplasia (an incidence of cancer/dysplasia of $9/55 = 16\%$); five patients had cancer discovered as a result of colonoscopic surveillance biopsies. It is highly likely that the finding of dysplasia in 11% of patients in the surveillance group will identify an ultra-high-risk category that must be more closely observed in the future. The low incidence of colon carcinoma associated with dysplasia in these studies may suggest that a combination of the patchy nature of dysplasia and the small amount of colon actually sampled on endoscopic biopsies weigh against the likelihood of a greater diagnostic yield. Because of the finding of carcinoma on direct endoscopic mucosal biopsy in an additional 1% (five of 479 patients) of patients in the high-risk group, a plea must be made that, in this category of patients with ulcerative colitis, more frequent rather than less frequent colonoscopies should be performed, allowing the opportunity for repeated multiple-area sampling, so that the subgroup with carcinoma or those at ultra-high risk for the development of carcinoma can be identified. Grandqvist [4] has demonstrated both the regression of dysplasia or the total absence of such findings on repeated colonoscopic biopsy. A single report of dysplasia on endoscopic biopsy should not result in the decision for surgery in the patient with chronic universal ulcerative colitis. If inflammation is also present, further biopsies should be taken after therapy of the disease; in the absence of inflammation, repeat biopsy must be obtained in 3–6 months, and colectomy should be performed only if dysplasia is persistently identified.

The number of ulcerative colitis patients in the high-risk group is not large, consisting of 479 patients being followed colonoscopically. Of these, 14 (11%) have been found to have cancer. The malignancies that are discovered via surveillance are usually early and curable. In order to identify these early neoplasms, it is suggested that colonoscopy be performed in the high-risk group yearly, and, if dysplasia is found, the examination should be repeated in 3–6 months.

Since ulcerative colitis is characteristically a disease with the most severe inflammatory areas located distally, the ability to biopsy proximal segments may permit more precise differentiation of dysplasia unhindered by inflammatory infiltrates. The use of a shorter 'flexible sigmoidoscope' permits biopsy of the left colon but provides only a limited addition to the area visualized with the proctosigmoidoscope. The use of this instrument has no role in the evaluation or endoscopic surveillance of patients with chronic ulcerative colitis.

Subtotal colectomies in patients with universal ulcerative colitis are performed for several reasons, one of which is the desire of both the patient and the surgeon eventually to re-establish bowel continuity with an ileorectal anastomosis. It is important to evaluate the degree of inflammation in the rectal segment prior to any such anastomosis. Frequently, the rectum becomes narrow following its bypass, and strictures may form just inside the anal canal. In these patients, sigmoidoscopy may be difficult but can be easily accomplished with the flexible fibreoptic endoscope, either standard-sized or paediatric. The presence of marked inflammation with pus, ulcerations and friability contraindicates re-anastomosis. However, it should be noted that disuse of the rectal segment may result in spontaneous friability of its mucosal surface, and biopsies must be taken to ascertain whether the mucosa is actually affected by the underlying colitis disease or is friable as a result of bypass disuse. Because of the propensity of carcinoma to develop within a retained rectal segment, every effort must be made to survey the rectal segment on a regular basis if reanastomosis is not accomplished.

SUMMARY

Colonoscopy offers little assistance in the surgical evaluation for most patients with ulcerative colitis. However, when used for well-defined goals, it may be of benefit in establishing the correct differential diagnosis between ulcerative and granulomatous colitis, in the evaluation of radiographic abnormalities, such as strictures and mass lesions, and in the diagnosis of cancer and premalignant changes in the colon. The great majority of strictures in patients with ulcerative colitis are benign and will not require operative intervention. The proper evaluation of strictures is outlined. Surveillance of the high-risk patient with ulcerative colitis should be accomplished on an annual basis, with more frequent examinations when dysplastic cells are discovered on colonoscopic biopsies.

REFERENCES

1. Glotzer, D. J. and Silen, W. (1981) in *Inflammatory Bowel Disease*, 2nd edn, (eds J. B. Kirsner and R. G. Shorter), Lea & Febiger, Phila., pp. 488–515.
2. Kirsner, J. B. (1980) Observations on the medical treatment of inflammatory bowel disease. *JAMA*, **243**, (6), 557–64.
3. Teague, R. H. and Waye, J. D. (1980) in *Colonoscopy*, (eds R. H. Hunt and J. D. Waye), Chapman and Hall Ltd., London, pp. 343–61.
4. Grandqvist, S., Gabrielsson, N., Sundelin, P. *et al.* (1980) Precancerous lesions in the mucosa in ulcerative colitis. A radiographic, endoscopic, and histopathologic study. *Scand. J. Gastroenterol.*, **15**, 289–96.
5. Williams, C. B. and Waye, J. D. (1978) Colonoscopy in inflammatory bowel disease. *Clin. Gastroenterol.*, **7**, 701–17.
6. Crespon, B., Housset, P., Mendez, J. *et al.* (1975) Bilan de 1000 colonoscopies. *Arch. Franc. Malad. Apparat. Dig.*, **64**, 229–308.
7. Fruhmorgen, P. (1974) Diagnosis of inflammatory bowel diseases of the colon by colonoscopy. *Acta Gastroenterol. Belgica*, **37**, 154–8.
8. Teague, R. H. and Waye, J. D. (1981) in *Colonoscopy: Techniques, Clinical Practice and Colour Atlas* (eds R. H. Hunt and J. D. Waye), Chapman and Hall, Ltd., London, pp. 343–62.
9. Teague, R. H. and Read, A. E. (1975) Polyposis in ulcerative colitis. *Gut*, **16**, 792–5.
10. Fitterer, J. D., Major M. C., Cromwell, L. G. *et al.* (1977) Colonic obstruction by giant pseudopolyposis. *Gastroenterology*, **72**, 153–6.
11. Dawson, I. M. and Pryse-Davies, J. (1959) The development of carcinoma of the large intestine in ulcerative colitis. *Br. J. Surg.*, **47**, 113–28.
12. Waye, J. D. and Hunt, R. H. (1982) Colonoscopic diagnosis of inflammatory bowel disease. *Surg. Clin. N. Am.*, **62**, 905–13.

13. Hunt, R. H., Teague, R. H., Swarbrick, E. T. *et al.* (1975) Colonoscopy in management of colonic strictures. *Br. Med. J.*, **2**, 360–1.
14. Waye, J. D. (1978) Colitis, cancer, and colonoscopy. *Med. Clin. N. Am.*, **62**, 211–24.
15. Crowson, T. D., Ferrante, W. F. and Cathright, J. B., Jr. (1976) Colonoscopy: inefficacy for early carcinoma detection in patients with ulcerative colitis. *JAMA*, **236**, 2651–2.
16. Morson, B. C. (1974) Evolution of cancer of the colon and rectum. *Cancer*, **34**, 845–9.
17. Morson, B. C. and Pang, L. S. (1967) Rectal biopsy as an aid to cancer control in ulcerative colitis. *Gut*, **8**, 423–34.
18. Nugent, F. W. and Haggitt, R. C. (1980) Long-term follow-up, including cancer surveillance, for patients with ulcerative colitis. *Clin. Gastroenterol.*, **9**, 459–76.
19. Riddell, R. H. and Morson, B. C. (1979) Value of sigmoidoscopy and biopsy in detection of carcinoma and premalignant change in ulcerative colitis. *Gut*, **20**, 575–80.
20. Riddell, R. H. (1977) Endoscopic recognition of early carcinoma in ulcerative colitis. *JAMA*, **237**, 2811.
21. Nugent, F. W., Haggitt, R. C., Colcher, H. *et al.* (1979) Malignant potential of chronic ulcerative colitis. *Gastroenterology*, **76**, 1–5.
22. Dobbins, W. O. (1977) Current status of the precancer lesion in ulcerative colitis. *Gastroenterology*, **73**, 1431–3.
23. Riddell, R. H. (1980) Dysplasia in inflammatory bowel disease. *Clin. Gastroenterol.*, **9**, 439–58.
24. Riddell, R. H. (1979) The precarcinomatous phase of ulcerative colitis. *Curr. Topic. Pathol.*, **63**, 179–219.
25. Dobbins, W. O., Stock, M. and Ginsberg, A. L. (1977) Early detection and prevention of carcinoma of the colon in patients with ulcerative colitis. *Cancer*, **40**, 2542–52.
26. Waye, J. D. (1980) in *Colorectal Cancer: Prevention, Epidemiology, and Screening* (eds S. Winawer, D. Schotenfeld, and P. Sherlock), Raven Press, New York, pp. 387–92.
27. Fuson, J. A., Farmer, R. G., Hawk, W. A. *et al.* (1980) Endoscopic surveillance for cancer in chronic ulcerative colitis. *Am. J. Gastroenterol.*, **73**, 120–6.
28. Dickinson, R. J., Dixon, M. F. and Axon, A. P. R. (1980) Colonoscopy and the detection of dysplasia in patients with long standing ulcerative colitis. *Lancet*, **ii**, 620–2.
29. Lennard-Jones, J. E., Morson, B. C., Path, F. R. *et al.* (1977) Cancer in colitis: assessment of the individual risk by clinical and histological criteria. *Gastroenterology*, **73**, 1280–9.
30. Blackstone, M. O., Riddell, R. H., Rogers, B. H. *et al.* (1980) Dysplasia-associated lesion or mass (DALM) detected by colonoscopy in long-standing ulcerative colitis: an indication for colectomy. *Gastroenterology*, **80**, 366–74.

23

In support of the colonoscopist: the pathologist

J. D. DAVIES

TUMOUR LIFE HISTORY

In recent years it has become evident that carcinomas have a longer life history than used to be thought. Although there are considerable variations in the growth rate of breast cancers [1], it is estimated that the slower growing carcinomas in the breast have been present for ten or more years before attaining palpable size [2]. A similar lengthy evolution of the polyp-cancer sequence in the large bowel has been postulated [3].

The implications of these observations are that there is a long time during which early diagnosis could be made. In most tissues, once stromal invasion has occurred the possibility of lymphatic or venous invasion exists. Skeletal scintigraphy has demonstrated that many apparent Stage I breast carcinomas have metastasized to the skeleton shortly after diagnosis of the primary tumour [4]. However, the absence of lymphatic vessels in the colorectal mucosa diminishes the chance of metastasis whilst the tumour remains confined to the colorectal lamina propria [5]. This situation contrasts with the establishment of metastases by gastric mucosal carcinoma.

Ideally, it could be argued that surgical resection of tumours should be performed whilst the lesions are still in their *in situ* phase before stromal invasion has occurred. Perhaps, carrying such considerations further it could be maintained that epidemiological and laboratory evidence should be utilized to eliminate the causative agents responsible for the cancer. However, we do not live in an ideal world and, alas, colorectal neoplasia seems likely to remain a part of the gastrointestinal and endoscopic scene for the forseeable future.

Experimental tumour models have indicated that potentially neoplastic cells may undergo a series of changes before expressing their neoplastic character [6].

The first change in some chemically-induced tumours appears to be initiation, followed by a more prolonged phase of promotion in which cellular proliferation occurs. Possibly, such a sequence only occurs in relatively few animal models, and there is some uncertainty as to how they correspond to events in human tumours. In morphological terms, initiation is unlikely to be recognizable for it may involve only one or at most only very few cells. The histological changes during promotion will certainly involve hyperplasia, or cellular proliferation. However it is not a process that morphologically is distinguishable from hyperplasia due to the many other stimuli which provoke cellular proliferation. Such early events in the development of tumours are not possible, at least with our current methods, to recognize in man. Equally, the precancerous significance of metaplasia, which is often a feature of epithelia at risk of cancer is not meaningful in an individual patient.

DYSPLASIA AND *IN SITU* CARCINOMA

If hyperplasia and metaplasia are too non-specific to lead to prognostication, what changes lead to real suspicion of tumour development? During the 1930s it became evident that surface and glandular epithelia in the vicinity of overt invasive carcinomas showed cytological and structural changes that bore a close resemblance to the invasive carcinomas [7, 8]. As a result, the concept of *in situ* or intramucosal carcinoma arose. This was, and still is, a clinical contradiction in terms, since it implies a characteristic which is clearly not fully expressed by the epithelium. Therapeutically, it carries the implication that, unless a wide field change is occurring, the radical surgery adopted for invasive cancer is inappropriate. Once attention was focused on the surface epithelium, it became clear that abnormal growth patterns which were not orderly hyperplasia, and yet not full-blown *in situ* carcinoma, were also demonstrable. It is these atypical hyperplasias, precancerous changes, which were later to be called dysplastic lesions [9]. Similar changes were also found in exfoliated cytological preparations from a variety of organs. Although different nomenclatures were adopted – with the expected resultant confusion – it is now generally accepted that such preparations show the same phenomenon which are to be seen in histological sections. Indeed in the organ most studied by exfoliative cytology, namely the cervix uteri, there is now fairly general agreement as to the correlation between cytological and histopathological changes.

Large national screening projects for cervical cancer have yielded much useful information about the behaviour of epithelial dysplasia, at least as it affects the cervix [10]. By virtue of the relatively small size of the cervix – allowing for complete examination by both cytological and histological means – and the varying fashions in the surgical treatment of such cervical lesions there is now a considerable body of evidence as to the behaviour of cervical dysplasia, *in situ* carcinoma and microinvasive carcinoma. The mean ages at which cervical dysplasia, *in situ* carcinoma and invasive carcinoma of cervix are found (whilst obviously subject to considerable individual variation) are suggestive of a progressive sequence. The resemblances to similar data available on postgastrectomy stumps and colorectal carcinoma arising in familial polyposis or ulcerative colitis in the years after the initial abnormality are obvious. However, at least in the cervix, it is clear that none of the degrees of dysplasia, or even *in situ* carcinoma, are necessarily progressive, since follow-up with serial biopsy or exfoliative cytology indicates that a substantial proportion of these lesions either regresses or does not progress [10].

A further complication is raised by the evidence that the behaviour of the cervical lesions is also influenced by the age of the patient. Possibly, this may relate to the fact that the incidence of cervical carcinoma does not continue to rise progressively after the fifth decade of life, unlike colorectal carcinoma which shows a progressive rise in incidence with increasing age. A linear relation to age is found when both age and incidence rates of colorectal cancer are plotted on a logarithmic scale, at least when the common types of colorectal carcinoma are considered [11].

GASTROINTESTINAL DYSPLASIAS

In moving to consider the stomach and large bowel it will be immediately obvious that there are considerable problems involved in the study of these organs if similar behaviour occurs in their mucosal epithelium. With the exception of colonic polyposis, and of isolated sigmoid or rectal adenomatous polyps, there used to be little opportunity for the morphologist to study the temporal development of dysplastic lesions in the colon and rectum. However, with the advent of the relatively recent art of endoscopy there are greater possibilities of morphological examination. Indeed by virtue of the ability to repeat endoscopic examination some idea of the progression, regression or static character of dysplasia may be gained. Clearly long-term studies must necessarily be in their infancy. Another difficulty is that of making complete examinations of gastric and colonic resections. Full blocking of a cervical cone is accomplished in 10–20 paraffin blocks. An entire stomach would require more than 200, and the number for a colorectal resection I leave to your imagination. Most pathologists, with the close collaboration of their endoscopists adopt a compromise in an attempt to study the particularly relevant areas of such organs [12]. Implicit in such examinations, of excised organs is the halt in the natural history of the very disease which we wish to study. It is this factor which makes it very difficult to devise any long-term follow-up on the more worrisome lesions which will be discussed later. My feeling is that currently we are not in the position of students of cervical dysplasia and *in situ* carcinoma, and necessarily do not have any means of following the natural history of these lesions in the colon and rectum after substantial resections. Endoscopy, by means of its limited biopsies, may allow for serial studies of dysplasia over a period of time. At least in the first instance, it seems that only relatively low-grade or dubious dysplasia will be studied in this way.

Not only are there deficiencies in the pathological study of dysplastic colorectal lesions, but we also lack the endoscopic facilities of the cervical gynaecologist. At present there does not exist an instrument with the power of resolution of a colposcope whereby the detailed vascular arrangement could be examined in colorectal mucosa. Possibly the vascular abnormalities, which might be related to release of a tumour angiogenetic factor [13], may help guide endoscopic biopsy to relevant, if otherwise unimpressive mucosal lesions.

The biological behaviour of dysplastic epithelium in the colon and rectum has been studied mainly by means of retrospective assessment of colorectal resections. In this manner correlations have been found between it and other frankly malignant tumours. Prospective studies of polyposis coli, isolated polyps, and inflammatory bowels with dysplasia have necessarily been less extensive. The situation corresponds to the early phases in the study of uterine cervical dysplasia. It is clear to those who are not directly concerned with the clinical management of patients with demonstrable dysplasia, that there is a natural reluctance to extend observations on the natural history of untreated dysplasia. This attitude reflects the known statistical inevitability of invasive carcinoma in untreated polyposis coli, and to the especially malignant character of cancer arising in ulcerative colitis. Extirpation of solitary or limited numbers of colorectal adenomas and their variants clearly interferes with the natural development of such lesions. For all these reasons there is a justifiable disinclination to embark upon a prospective study of the unmodified natural history of large bowels bearing dysplastic lesions. Currently, surgical opinion does not allow the varied approach to these lesions, which is in practice adopted for *in situ* lobular neoplasia of the breast. Probably until there is better evidence that subsets of colorectal dysplastic lesions have a relatively benign course it is unlikely that many clinicians will be reconciled to a wait-and-see policy with the more severe of these lesions.

In any single unit cases of dysplasia arising in inflammatory bowel disease are relatively few, and hence tend to be regarded with great suspicion. Data on such cases are necessarily limited but the risk of an associated carcinoma in a patient with total colitis is considerable, as has been reviewed in the preceding paper. In diagnostic histological practice, my personal suspicion is that pathologists, knowing of the likely surgical steps that may result from an unequivocal diagnosis of any form of dysplasia, tend to ignore or at least underplay the changes that constitute the lesser degrees of atypical hyperplasia or dysplasia. Such a state of affairs is regrettable if an attempt is being made to make an objective analysis of the natural history of dysplastic lesions. A similar underdiagnosis by pathologists of alcoholic cirrhosis – in this case prompted by the forensic implications – may have been responsible for the only comparatively recent acceptance of how frequent alcohol-associated cirrhosis is in England and Wales.

New international definition of colorectal dysplasia

The dual problems of framing an acceptable morphological definition, and then of achieving its widespread acceptance, are clearly interrelated. Fortunately, in the case of colorectal dysplasia arising in inflammatory bowel disease, these difficulties seem likely to be solved shortly. An international group of colorectal pathologists have been meeting at intervals to investigate the topic. This team, coordinated by Dr J. H. Yardley of Baltimore, has recently presented their findings in a poster demonstration at a meeting of the American Gastroenterological Association in New York. That display, with the associated photomicrographs, is available from several of the members of the group (Morson, B. C., personal communication).

It seems likely that this group will be able to provide workable morphological definitions of the grades of colorectal dysplasia. Their experience and reputation should ensure acceptance of their proposals. A further potential advantage of their classification is that it is soundly based upon the subsequent clinical management of the lesions.

To a pathologist one of the main virtues of the method adopted by Yardley's panel is that they are using an ongoing means of reaching their morphological definitions. In the case of cervical dysplasia reasonably firm definitions of the changes were extant before they were submitted to the pathological audits, of the type described by Ringsted et al. [14]. The evolving Yardley-group definition is being evaluated in these terms during its formation. As one actively involved in a similar exercise in dysplastic breast lesions studied on a national basis, their approach seems to me a distinct advance upon the empirical morphological definitions of earlier days.

As yet, the details of this group's definitions of colorectal dysplasia in inflammatory bowel disease have not been published. Pathologists involved in the field eagerly await the results of this important investigation, and will welcome a classification already submitted to such an internal audit. To many, it seems disappointing that other internationally-based classifications of tumours in other organs are not developed in a like manner.

PATHOLOGICAL CONSISTENCY

The approach adopted by Yardley's team leads to the consideration of the serious deficiency in the ability of the histopathologist to make a consistent assessment of dysplastic lesions. Morphological diagnosis is no less complex than clinical diagnosis [15, 16]. It is partly based upon a combination of preconceived theoretical considerations and of the analysis of a complex series of microscopic changes. In the occasional case histopathological diagnosis depends upon lateral thinking and the process of linking anomalous features to make an apparently unexpected diagnosis. Most histopathological diagnosis is not of that character, and depends upon assessment of a relatively limited number of changes, which are apparently easily encapsulated in definitions. Such routine diagnoses are seemingly easily transmitted to inexperienced trainee pathologists, and universally incorporated in practical examinations designed to test the competence of young pathologists. In a sense, the diagnosis of the sequence of changes ranging from mild dysplasia through *in situ* carcinoma to invasive carcinoma is a good example of the type of lesion which it is hoped that the experienced histopathologist could adequately train his juniors to recognize and to categorize.

Surprisingly it is only in the last few years that any attempt has been made by pathologists to see whether such training is effective. Probably most clinicians have long had their own suspicions, and may even have initiated private experiments on these lines! One of my reasons for introducing the topic of cervical dysplastic lesions is that this is one of the fields in which the earliest systemic attempt to assess the consistency of assessment of dysplastic lesions was made. The results were, at first sight sufficiently startling as to justify the feeling of many experimental pathologists that methods other than those of morphology are preferable. Quantiative analysis by means of biochemistry, cytofluorimetry, or by using any measurable parameter is a well established principle in experimental pathology. Personally I think that this was an over-reaction for reasons that will become evident later in this discussion.

However, a Danish department of pathology circulated 1001 sections of cervical biopsy sections for assessment by four 'experienced' and nine trainee pathologists [14]. The histological assessments of the individual pathologists is shown in Table 23.1 in relation to the consensus assessment by three of the 'experienced' pathologists. From a practical point of view the likelihood of a 'correct' diagnosis being reached by an individual is shown in Table 23.2. The excellent training in

Table 23.1 Array of diagnoses made by ordinary and experienced pathologists of cervical lesions

Ordinary diagnosis	Peer diagnosis				
	1	2	3	4	5
(1) Normal	6576	205	128	32	12
(2) Mild dysplasia	256	112	139	23	2
(3) Severe dysplasia	50	62	299	112	10
(4) Carcinoma *in situ*	11	3	97	216	16
(5) Invasive carcinoma	11	2	5	12	495

Data from Ringsted *et al.* [14]

Table 23.2 Probabilities of diagnosis of cervical lesions

	Diagnosis probabilities (%)				
Ordinary diagnosis	1	2	3	4	5
(1) Normal	94	3	2	<1	<1
(2) Mild dysplasia	49	21	26	4	<1
(3) Severe dysplasia	9	12	56	21	2
(4) Carcinoma *in situ*	3	1	28	63	5
(5) Invasive carcinoma	2	<1	1	2	94

Data from Ringsted *et al.* [14]

this particular department is shown by the finding that although trainee pathologists showed an increased variation in their subsequent diagnostic attempts (an assessment of intraobserver error), as opposed to their seniors, in fact their departure from the consensus diagnosis was not statistically different from that exhibited by the staff members (interobserver error).

Similar variations have subsequently been demonstrated amongst highly experienced and interested pathologists participating in a similar assessment of dysplastic breast lesions, and amongst the pathologists of international repute mentioned above in assessing colorectal biopsy lesions in which dysplasia was assessed.

At first sight the percentage probabilities of a 'correct' or 'consensus' diagnosis from individuals are less than reassuring to the clinician. However there are features which are common to all three series and are not so alarming from a practical aspect. The least agreement in diagnostic assessment is met in the 'grey' zones wherein degrees of dysplasia are being graded. Secondly such exercises have highlighted the fact that often an individual pathologist is groping for an ill-defined concept of what constitutes the divisions between these intermediate categories of dysplasia. These definitions have been amazingly little discussed either in formal communications or in day-to-day discussion between colleagues. One notable exception, happily in the field of dysplasia in inflammatory bowel disease, demonstrates the virtues of an open airing of the difficulties encountered [17]. The extensive discussion in that symposium illustrates the variety of views as to what constitutes colorectal dysplasia, and how it should be graded. This type of difficulty is one that is acknowledged by most pathologists who are prepared to express their concern about such matters. Nonetheless it has remained, until recently, a covert and insufficiently discussed topic. One hopes that such attempts to reveal the character of the problem will reassure others that it is a basic and universal difficulty in the assessment of the lesions which appear to be potential precursors of overt malignancy.

METHODS OF IMPROVED PATHOLOGICAL DIAGNOSIS

How may such problems be resolved? In part, it is to be hoped that the results of more investigations into histopathological consistency will be published, if only to reassure those pathologists who hold unspoken fears of their own performance in this field. Such revelations are likely to stimulate attempts to improve consistency in diagnostic performance.

The improvements are likely to follow two developments. The first, and simplest, is the framing of more precise criteria for the categories of dysplasia. Such definitions may be improved by the application of modern methods of stereology or quantitative analysis of microscopic images. The second is related to the vectorial or cluster analysis, already well known to clinicians interested in the diagnosis of inflammatory bowel disease. Such methods are now being applied to the analysis of morphological appearances.

Morphological criteria of dysplasia

Criteria of dysplasia and its various stages are clearly the subject of considerable histological debate. There have been made proposals for the definition of mild, moderate and severe dysplasia [17]. Illustrative examples are very helpful to pathologists in allocating a given lesion to one of these categories. However, even the help given by this method, still leaves problems in 'correct' assignation of borderline lesions. In many organs new patterns of dysplastic growth are constantly being recognized, which add further confusion to the field. Most of the criteria of dysplasia mainly stress cytological features and the polarity of the arrangement of the epithelial cells. Even at this level there still remain the difficulties of framing a sufficiently precise morphological definition, and of gaining its general acceptance. Thereafter the pathologist in the field has the exercise of matching images in order to grade the type of dysplasia.

In addition to individual cellular features, and the polar arrangement of the epithelium, the growth pattern of the units containing the cells merits consideration. The glands of the stomach and endometrium in states of dysplasia often exhibit increased branching. The branching may become so complex that it is virtually impossible to know from sectioned material when detachment and stromal invasion first commences. Judgements on these changes will necessarily be subjective. Recently quantitative morphological methods have been applied to these lesions [18]. The results suggest that stereological analysis may give an objective support to the subjective interpretation by the hisopathologist. The virtues of the method are that it is more reliable, and capable of quantitating a continuum of changes.

Although the presence of stromal invasion by colorectal epithelial neoplasms may have less serious implications than in other organs, a similar stereological approach may contribute to the grading of colorectal dysplasia. Currently there is considerable development in commercial quantitative image-analysis systems. It is true that they are extremely expensive, but it will be of interest to see whether further advances in technology will allow such methods to become feasible for routine use. A possible solution may be found in the establishment of reference centres to deal with the morphological analysis. Certainly this may raise logistic problems in the clinical management of cases, and it would seem preferable for the image analysis to take place in the laboratory where the conventional assessments were taking place. It is likely that such analytical methods may help reframe the definitions of dysplasia, or supplement those directed to subjective assessment.

On a less theoretical plane, other features in a biopsy may modify the interpretation of the epithelial changes outlined above. Regenerating or actively inflamed epithelium may acquire the morphology seen in mild and moderate, and possibly, some types of severe dysplasia. A background of severe active inflammation is usually held to preclude a diagnosis of dysplasia.

Vectorial analysis of morphology

Vectorial analysis of morphological appearances is an analytical method which helps the recognition of helpful discriminating features in diagnosis. It has been employed in the study of borderline malignant lesions of the oral mucosa [19], and might help in the definition of colorectal dysplasia. Fundamentally the method involves study of a range of previously determined morphological components in lesions. Subsequent multidimensional analysis reveals which morphological features prove to be helpful discriminants to separate diagnostic categories. Such a method may highlight features which are only dimly appreciated as having some association with the main lesion under study. Equally it can be helpful in analysing features which are usually accepted as being intrinsic to the category being diagnosed. Later analysis can show in a quantitative manner whether such assumptions are justified. Naturally with computer facilities it is possible to combine this approach with that of automatic quantitative image analysis. Using the extended range of data generated by image analysis it is likely that this type of multidimensional will indicate which features are of useful discriminant value. As immunohistochemistry evolves, its place, too, may be subjected to the same method of evaluation.

The main advantage that these modern approaches offers is that in restricted fields they obviate the need for inspired or subconscious methods of diagnosis by the histopathologist. Even in the relatively limited problem posed to the morphologist by dysplasia, it is clear from the results of consistency surveys that currently the pathologist is not an entirely reliable interpreter. An quantitative analysis, aided by multidimensional statistical evaluation appears a remote and academic activity. However, the results of such investigations could well aid the routine diagnostic pathologist faced by possible or overt dysplasia. Perhaps future work may highlight relatively readily graded components in the lesions, which would aid accurate and reproducible grading of dysplasia.

In order to institute appropriate clinical management there is an urgent need for a suitable classification of dysplasia in inflammatory bowel disease. The approach adopted by Yardley's group has the advantage that it is firmly directed towards such clinical implications. Its additional virtue is the incorporation of an internal audit during its development, which should help improve the consistency with which other pathologists can apply it. If such a classification is widely used the number of cases of consistently graded dysplasia in inflammatory bowel disease will be greatly increased. This will allow the possibility of studying the behaviour of the graded lesions. Obviously, the large surface area of the colorectal mucosa makes for difficulty in endoscopic and pathological examination. Such an anatomical factor offers more problems than those posed by the uterine cervix. However, the combination of endoscopy and consistent pathological grading of dysplasia in inflammatory bowel disease seems likely to lead towards answering the questions that have been posed of cervical dysplasia in the recent times.

SUMMARY

The historical development of the concept of epithelial dysplasia is outlined. The behaviour of dysplasia in the cervix suggests that progression to carcinoma may not be inevitable. The comparative states of study of colorectal and cervical dysplasia are described. The continuous spectrum of changes in dysplasia lead to difficulties in its grading. Consistency of pathological assessment of dysplasia in inflammatory bowel disease is a necessity before appropriate clinical management can be instituted. Ways in which consistency can be achieved are discussed with particular reference to morphological definition, pathological auditing, quantitative image processing and multidimensional statistical analysis.

ACKNOWLEDGEMENTS

I am grateful to colleagues in many disciplines for discussions of the methods described in this paper. My thanks are also due to Miss V. A. Thyer for typing the manuscript.

REFERENCES

1. Heuser, L., Spratt, J. S. and Polk, H. C. (1979) Growth rates of primary breast cancers. *Cancer*, **43**, 1888–94.
2. Haagensen, C. D. (ed) (1971) *Disease of The Breast*, Saunders, Philadelphia, p. 383.

3. Muto, T., Bussey, H. J. R. and Morson, B. C. (1975) The evolution of cancer of the colon and rectum. *Cancer*, **36**, 2251–70.
4. Galasko, C. S. P. (1969) The detection of skeletal metastases from mammary cancer by gamma camera scintigraphy. *Br. J. Surg.*, **56**, 757–64.
5. Morson, B. C. and Dawson, I. M. P. (eds) (1979) *Gastrointestinal Pathology*, 2nd edn, Blackwell, Oxford, p. 609.
6. Medline, A. and Farber, E. (1981) in *Recent Advances in Histopathology*, No. 11, (eds P. P. Anthony and R. N. M. MacSween), Churchill-Livingstone, Edinburgh, pp. 19–34.
7. Broders, A. C. (1932) Carcinoma *in situ* contrasted with benign penetrating epithelium. *J. Am. Med. Assoc.*, **99**, 1670–4.
8. Muir, R. (1941) The evolution of carcinoma of the mamma. *J. Pathol. Bactol.*, **52**, 155–72.
9. Reagan, J. W., Seidermann, I. L. and Saracusa, Y. (1953) Cellular morphology of carcinoma-*in situ* and dysplasia or atypical hyperplasia of the uterine cervix. *Cancer*, **6**, 224–35.
10. Langley, F. A. and Crompton, A. C. (1973) Epithelial abnormalities of the cervix uteri. *Rec. Res. Canc. Res.*, **40**.
11. Miller, D. G. (1980) On the nature of susceptibility to cancer. *Cancer*, **46**, 1307–18.
12. Davies, J. D., Tudway, A. J. C., Roberts, G. and Machado, G. (1976) Detection of superficial gastric carcinoma in biopsies and resected stomachs. *J. Clin. Pathol.*, **29**, 756–7.
13. Folkman, J., Merler, E., Abernathy, C. and Williams, G. (1971) Isolation of a tumor factor responsible for angiogenesis. *J. Exp. Med.*, **133**, 275–88.
14. Ringsted, J. *et al.* (1978) Reliability of histo-pathological diagnosis of squamous epithelial changes of the uterine cervix. *Acta Pathol. Microbiol. Scand. (Sect. A)*, **86**, 273–8.
15. King, L. S. (1967) How does a pathologist make a diagnosis? *Arch. Pathol.*, **84**, 331–3.
16. Underwood, J. C. E. (1981) *Introduction to Biopsy Interpretation and Surgical Pathology.* Springer-Verlag, Berlin.
17. Fenoglio, C. M., Haggitt, R. C., Hamilton, S. R., Lumb, G. *et al.* (1981) Colonic dysplasia (a symposium). *Pathol. Ann.*, **16** (I), 181–213.
18. Bach, J. P. A., Kurver, P. H. J., Diegenbach, P. C., Delemarre, J. F. M. *et al.* (1981) Discrimination of hyperplasia and carcinoma of the endometrium by quantitative microscopy – a feasibility study. *Histopathology*, **5**, 61–8.
19. Kramer, I. R. H., El-Labban, N. G. and Sonkodi, S. (1974) Further studies on lesions of the oral mucosa using computer-aided analyses of histological features. *Br. J. Canc.*, **29**, 223–31.

Index